STYLE GUIDE
FOR MEDICAL TRANSCRIPTION

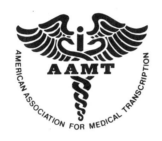

by

Claudia Tessier, CMT, RRA
M.Ed., Allied Health
Director of Education

Sally C. Pitman, CMT
M.A., English
Director of Publications

AMERICAN ASSOCIATION FOR MEDICAL TRANSCRIPTION

1985

©1985 by American Association for Medical Transcription, Modesto, California. All rights reserved.

American Association for Medical Transcription
A Nonprofit Professional Corporation
P. O. Box 6187, Modesto, California 95355
Phone 209-576-0883, 800-982-2182, 800-624-4924.

Last digit is the print number: 9   8   7   6   5   4   3

Design, layout, photocomposition by Prima Vera Publications, Modesto, California.

Printing and binding by Riverbank Printing Company, Riverbank, California.

*To
Vera Pyle,
who began the dialogue
on Style*

ACKNOWLEDGMENTS

This book could not have been written without the assistance of hundreds, even thousands, of medical transcriptionists. Among them are the thousand medical transcriptionists who attended the AAMT Exploring Transcription Practices workshops in 1983 and 1984; their interest and desire to learn and understand and to improve their skills were major stimulants for the preparation of this book. Hundreds more have called or written the American Association for Medical Transcription, asking questions that confirmed for us the need for a compilation of stylistic guidelines. And still hundreds more have approached us at the AAMT annual meetings seeking information and clarification on transcription practices. Mention must also be made of students and trainees, co-workers and colleagues who planted the seeds of thought which eventually led to the preparation of the *Style Guide.*

We also want to express our gratitude to those who served as manuscript reviewers for the *Style Guide:* Linda Campbell, Sue Covel, Karen Fields, Patricia Forbis, Patricia Horn, Avril Meehan, Vera Pyle, and Anne Shortridge. They painstakingly read the manuscript and offered corrections, alternatives, suggestions, and examples. Like the references we used in preparing the book, they differed among themselves and with us in certain matters; sometimes they changed our opinions, sometimes we changed theirs, and sometimes we agreed to disagree. In any case, we thank them for their time, effort, and encouragement.

Finally, we are grateful to the American Association for Medical Transcription for making it all possible.

PREFACE

The *Style Guide for Medical Transcription* is the result of many forces—some direct, others indirect. Naturally, our personal experiences as medical transcriptionists contributed, as did related activities such as teaching medical transcription and preparing educational materials and publications for the American Association for Medical Transcription.

We have been writing the *Style Guide* for years in our minds, but it wasn't until we developed and administered the AAMT Exploring Transcription Practices workshops in 1983 and 1984 that we began the actual documentation process. And the workshops provided the crucial direct link to medical transcriptionists with whom we could explore the styles, content, and practices of medical transcription. Because the workshops involved meeting with our peers, we knew we had to be able to explain every detail of the transcripts to be discussed. It wouldn't be enough to say, "I've always done it this way"; we had to be able to explain why.

So we opened all the references we've been using for years, as well as many new ones, and began the documentation search. As word-search addicts, we easily extended the habit to style, content, and usage research. The bibliography provided with the *Style Guide* demonstrates the lengths to which we went.

Sometimes the references agreed with us, other times they disagreed—not only with us but among themselves. It wasn't unusual for us to find improvements over longtime preferences, and we have changed some of our styles and practices as a result of the workshops and research for this book. We learned that in many instances there are *alternative acceptable* forms and styles in reporting medical data, and many of these are reflected here.

Findings through research were supplemented by our discussions with medical transcriptionists during the transcription workshops. We learned about new references and were reacquainted with old. Most significantly, we learned what medical transcriptionists were doing on the job, and what their questions and concerns were. More than any other AAMT activity in which we have engaged, the workshops provided the unique opportunity to "talk shop" with medical transcriptionists, and the use of real transcripts provided concrete examples as the basis of discussion. Some of these examples are repeated in the *Style Guide*; they are supplemented by examples from transcripts in the AAMT general medicine training module and other transcripts. Using examples from real dictation makes this a truly unique reference.

The workshops, in their preparation and delivery, demanded that we question ourselves and others and even the references, as has the preparation of the AAMT general medicine training module. Both experiences required that we acknowledge acceptable variations where they exist. They and the *Style Guide* preparation required that we reach conclusions—not ultimate conclusions, but sufficiently formed conclusions that we would be willing to share them with more than a thousand workshop participants and to put them into print to share with thousands more.

We don't expect all transcriptionists to agree with all of our conclusions. But we do expect that the *Style Guide* will make those who read it and use it think about their own practices, styles, and preferences.

As authors, editors, and professional colleagues, some of our greatest learning experiences have come about through discussions of our greatest differences (of which there are many). We challenge one another, and we want this book to challenge you. If you reach different conclusions, tell us what they are and why. This first *Style Guide for Medical Transcription* will lead to revisions and new editions, for which your input is essential.

Let the dialogue continue.

Claudia Tessier
Sally C. Pitman
December 1984

CONTENTS

ABBREVIATIONS

Approved abbreviations: Each hospital is required by the Joint Commission on Accreditation of Hospitals (JCAH) to prepare a list of acceptable abbreviations. Only abbreviations on that list should appear in that hospital's medical records. Hospital transcriptionists should have access to their hospital's list of approved abbreviations.

Do not use abbreviations (even those on the approved list) in admission diagnoses and impressions, discharge diagnoses, preoperative and postoperative diagnoses, and the names of operations and procedures.

    Dictated: Operation performed: TAH BSO.
    Transcribed: Operation performed: Total abdominal hysterectomy,
                                   bilateral salpingo-oophorectomy.

Elsewhere in medical reports, approved abbreviations may be used *if dictated.* Alternatively, dictated approved abbreviations may be written out in full. Do not use dictated abbreviations which are not on the approved list. If you are unable to translate the abbreviation, either type the abbreviation as dictated or leave a blank; in either case, flag the report to identify an unfamiliar abbreviation and ask its meaning.

Terminology dictated in full should **not** be abbreviated **except** for units of measurement. While the physician may dictate "milligrams," "centimeters," etc., the preferred form is to use the abbreviations (mg, cm, etc.); such abbreviations are universally known and accepted.

Medical slang: Medical slang and jargon must be avoided. See "Medical Slang—Its Use and Abuse," by Vera Pyle, in "A Question of Style," *Journal of the American Association for Medical Transcription,* Vol. 2, No. 3 (Fall 1983), pp. 38-39.

If slang terms are dictated, translate them in full in medical reports.

    Dictated: H. flu   Transcribed: H. influenzae
    Dictated: dex   Transcribed: dexamethasone
    Dictated: temp   Transcribed: temperature
    Dictated: lytes   Transcribed: electrolytes
    Dictated: appy   Transcribed: appendectomy

At beginning of sentence: Do not begin a sentence with an abbreviation.

    Dictated: WBC was 9200.
    Transcribed: White blood count was 9200.
               or: The WBC was 9200.

Capitalized abbreviations: Capitalize most abbreviations which are formed from selected letters of the word or phrase abbreviated. These abbreviations are called *initialisms* when they are formed from the first letters of each word. Do not use periods. Form the plural by adding **s.** While it is preferred to omit the apostrophe between the abbreviation and the **s,** it is acceptable to include it.

    BUS   Bartholin's, urethral, and Skene's glands

CABG	coronary artery bypass graft
CEA	carcinoembryonic antigen
CPK	creatine phosphokinase
ECG, EKG	electrocardiogram
EDC	estimated date of confinement
HEENT	head, eyes, ears, nose, and throat
IM	intramuscular
IV	intravenous
IU	international units
PMI	point of maximal impulse

Preferred:	PVCs	ABGs
Acceptable:	PVC's	ABG's

Acronyms: Capitalize all of the letters in *acronyms* (words composed of the initial letters of successive words in a phrase which may be pronounced as a word); do not use periods.

ECHO virus	enteric cytopathic human orphan virus
FANA	fluorescent antinuclear antibody
MAST	military antishock treatment
PERRLA	pupils equal, round, reactive to light and accommodation
SOAP	subjective, objective, assessment, plan

Some acronyms are so commonly used that they have become accepted as words which do not require translation; do not capitalize these and do not use periods.

laser   radar   rem   dopa

fabere sign   fadir sign

Lowercase abbreviations: The preferred style is to lowercase abbreviations used in relationship to the dosage or directions for medications, and to use periods. For other lowercase abbreviations, omit the periods; form the plural by adding an apostrophe and an **s.**

t.i.d.   p.o.   q.a.m.   p.r.n.   q.6h. or q. 6 h.

wbc, wbc's   rbc, rbc's

Mixed uppercase and lowercase abbreviations: Do not use periods in abbreviations which include uppercase and lowercase letters.

aVL   aVF   mEq   HbAg   iPTH   IgA   pH

Brief forms: Brief forms of words should not be followed by a period, unless the brief form may be misread as a different word. Do not capitalize brief forms unless the full form is capitalized. Form the plural by adding **s.** Do not use an apostrophe to form the plural. Avoid brief forms which are not generally acceptable. Use brief forms only if dictated.

ab	abortus, abortion
exam	examination
lap	laparotomy

Pap	Papanicolaou
preop	preoperative
postop	postoperative
prep	prepare
prepped	prepared (*prep'd* is *not* acceptable)
sed rate	sedimentation rate
subcu	subcutaneous, subcuticular (use abbreviation when it is unclear which meaning is intended)

but: in. (not *in* for inch)

Latin abbreviations: The abbreviations for certain Latin phrases, namely, **i.e.** (that is), **e.g.** (for example), **et al.** (and others), **etc.** (and so forth), are occasionally used in medical dictation. They are considered parenthetical, and for clarity a comma should be placed before and after each one used within a sentence.

The functional class may be preceded by a title, e.g., cardiac class or prognosis.

Ampersand: Avoid using the ampersand (&) except in phrases containing abbreviations separated by **and.** Do not space before or after the ampersand.

D&C	dilatation and curettage
T&A	tonsillectomy and adenoidectomy
A&P	auscultation and percussion; also, anterior and posterior (repair)

Abbreviations with numerals: Do not separate abbreviations from their associated numerals; i.e., type the figure and abbreviation on the same line. Space between the numeral and the abbreviation.

5700 WBC   47 mg%   35 mm   a dose of 0.8 mg/kg/hr.

Abbreviations with per: When expressing **per** with a slash, diagonal, or virgule (/), abbreviate associated units of measure.

Sed rate was noted to be 51 mm/hr.
not:
Sed rate was noted to be 51 millimeters/hour.

only 1 wbc/cu mm   or   1 wbc/mm^3
not:
only one white blood cell/cubic millimeter

Chemical symbols: Never use periods or hyphens with symbols for chemical elements or compounds.

O2   CO2   K   Na   FeSO4

Abbreviation mmHg: Use the abbreviation **mmHg** when the phrase "millimeters of mercury" is used in expressing pressure readings, e.g., blood pressure, tourniquet pressure. If the phrase is not dictated, the use of the abbreviation is optional.

Blood pressure 70/100.
Blood pressure 70/100 mmHg.

The tourniquet was inflated to 500 mmHg pressure.

Abbreviation pH: The pH of urine, blood, or other solution designates its alkalinity or acidity. The pH is expressed by a whole number or a whole number followed by a decimal point and one or two digits. The abbreviation **pH** must always be written with a lowercase p and uppercase H; do not use periods after the letters or a space between them. If a sentence starts with the abbreviation **pH,** insert the word "The" before it.

Dictated: pH was 4.5.
Transcribed: The pH was 4.5.

Units of measure: Do not abbreviate English or metric units of measure unless they are accompanied by a quantity. If the quantity is written out, as at the beginning of a sentence, then the unit of measure must also be written out. Always use a singular verb with units of measure.

Twenty milliequivalents of potassium chloride was given.
The patient was given 20 mEq of KCl.

Units of measure with quantities: When an abbreviation is used for a unit of measure, express the quantity by a numeral. If the unit of measure is written in full, the quantity may be expressed as a figure or written in full. Space between the numeral and the abbreviation.

5 mg, *not* five mg
8 in., *not* eight in.
five milligrams, 5 milligrams, or 5 mg

Metric units of measure: Abbreviations of metric units of measure with quantities are generally written in lowercase letters. Exception: Most abbreviations derived from proper names have an initial capital letter. Consult references for guidance. The abbreviation for **liter** may be written in lowercase or uppercase. Never use periods with abbreviations of units of measure in the metric system. Never use an **s** to form the plural of an abbreviation for a unit of measure.

5 mg	2 gm or g
10 cm	3.2 ng
15 cc	3 mm
Hz	W
Ci (or c)	l (or L)

English units of measure: The use of abbreviations for English units of measure with quantities is optional. When such abbreviations are used in medical reports, the use of periods is preferred but optional unless the abbreviation may be misread if the period is not used. Never use an **s** to form the plural of an abbreviation for a unit of measure.

Preferred: pound or lb., foot or ft.
Acceptable: lb, ft

but: inch or in., *not* in   8 in., *not* 8 in or 8 ins

Temperature readings: When expressing temperature readings, add the degree sign or the word **degrees** and F or C (for Fahrenheit or Celsius) if dictated; they are optional if not dictated. If the keyboard provides the degree sign (°), it is preferable to use it rather than writing out the word **degrees.**

35.4° *or* 35.4°C *or* 35.4 degrees
98.6° *or* 98.6°F *or* 98.6 degrees

Dates: It is preferred that dates be written in full in medical reports to assure clarity and accuracy. Avoid abbreviating the month or year or substituting the number of the month for its name. Write the day of the month as a number, either placing it before or after the month. In the month-day-year format (March 9, 1984) within a sentence, a comma must be placed after the day and also after the year.

Preferred: March 9, 1984, or 9 March 1984, or March 1984

Avoid: Mar 9 '84   3/9/84   3-9-84   9 Mar '84

The patient was seen in the office on March 9, 1984, after a three-day illness.

The patient was seen twice in March 1984 and admitted to the hospital on April 10.

The day may be expressed as an ordinal if so dictated and the year is not given. Do not use the ordinal form if the year is given.

March 20th (*not* March 20th, 1984)

Spell out the days of the week.

The patient will be seen in my office Tuesday, November 20.

Geographic names: Spell out the names of states, territories, or possessions of the United States within medical reports. Use abbreviations only in addresses, where they should be accompanied by zip codes. Spell out street addresses, including such words as Avenue, Street, Drive, and Lane. Exception: The abbreviations for directions (N, S, E, W, NW, NE, SE, and SW) are acceptable in addresses.

The patient has resided at 1538 Rodeo Drive, Orlando, Florida, for ten years.

Spell out the names of countries. Exception: The abbreviation USSR is acceptable for the Soviet Union.

The patient returned from Great Britain two weeks ago.

Genus name: Do not abbreviate a genus name the first time it is used in a report. It may be subsequently abbreviated provided it is dictated as an abbreviation and is accompanied by a species name.

Escherichia coli   *then* E. coli
Hemophilus influenzae   *then* H. influenzae

Species name: Do not abbreviate the species name when it is used in conjunction with the genus.

H. influenzae, *not* H. flu

Social titles: Always abbreviate social titles when used with the full name or surname. Drop these titles if another title is used.

Dr. Dirckx
Ms. Sue Covel
Mrs. Judith Marshall
Mr. Leon Pitman
Armand Brodeur, MD,   *not* Dr. Armand Brodeur, MD

Degrees or professional certification: The use of periods with abbreviations for degrees or professional certification is variable, and the trend is to omit them. Do not space between the letters of the abbreviation. When periods are used, do not space after them, except the final one. Place a comma after the individual's name and before the abbreviation.

James Bennington, MD	*or*	James Bennington, M.D.
Rita Finnegan, RRA	*or*	Rita Finnegan, R.R.A.
Anne Shortridge, CMT	*or*	Anne Shortridge, C.M.T.
Shirley Billups, RN	*or*	Shirley Billups, R.N.
Norman Billups, PhD, RPh	*or*	Norman Billups, Ph.D., R.Ph.

Initials of personal names: In initials of personal names, place a period after each initial, followed by a single space.

W. B. Saunders, *not* W.B. Saunders or WB Saunders

Business or organization names: Abbreviations for company names, associations, government agencies, service organizations, etc., are usually expressed in all capitals with no periods. Follow the preference of the organization in question.

AAMT, *not* A.A.M.T.
AMA, *not* A.M.A.
VA, *not* V.A.

Saint: The word **Saint** (abbreviated **St.**), when forming part of a personal or geographic name or the name of a health care institution, is written out or abbreviated according to the preference of the individual, place, or institution.

Mary St. James
Saint Mary's Hospital
Saint Mary Medical Center
St. Joseph Medical Clinic
St. Louis, Missouri

Use the abbreviation **St.** with names of operations, incisions, and instruments.

St. Clair forceps   St. Luke retractor

Dictator and transcriptionist initials: Type the dictator's and transcriptionist's initials at the end of a medical report or letter. Do not use periods and do not include titles. Depending on the style of the institution or the dictating physician, the dictator's initials precede those of the transcriptionist and either a colon or a slash may separate them.

RH:rs or RH/rs or rh:rs

APOSTROPHES

Time span: Use an apostrophe when expressing a time span in a possessive phrase.   Use a hyphen but no apostrophe when expressing a time span in a descriptive phrase.

a month's history (history of a month)   *but:* a one-month history
a few months' time (time of a few months)
an hour's delay   *but:* a one-hour delay
a two weeks' vacation   *but:* a two-week vacation
followup in three days' time   *but:* a three-day period

Contractions: Avoid contractions as much as possible in medical transcription; they make a formal, professional document look casual and informal.

Dictated: He's feeling much better.
Transcribed: He is feeling much better.

Dictated: It's unclear whether . . .
Transcribed: It is unclear whether . . .

Possession: For words not ending in **s**, show possession by adding an apostrophe and **s** (**'s**). For words ending in **s**, show possession by adding an apostrophe after the **s** (**s'**).

children's hospital
women's clinic
men's ward
few months' time
Physicians' Desk Reference
The patient's review of systems was noncontributory.
The species' identity has not yet been determined.

Possessive pronoun its: Do not use an apostrophe to form **its,** the possessive form of **it.** (The word **it's** is the contraction of **it is.** See **Contractions.**)

Its previous state was markedly changed.
It's (it is) too late to institute new measures.

Possessive eponyms: With eponyms followed by a noun, there is variable use of the possessive form for diseases, syndromes, tests, reflexes, operations, etc. Consult *Dorland's, Stedman's,* or *Current Medical Information & Terminology,* or use the dictating physician's preference. NOTE: If one of the articles **a, an** or **the** precedes the eponym, do **not** use an apostrophe to show possession. If the possessive form is used, follow the above rule, **Possession.**

> Abbe-Estlander operation
> Achilles tendon
> Bell's palsy
> Billroth's operation, *but* Billroth I operation
> Brudzinski's reflex
> Colles fracture
> Coombs' test
> Crohn's disease
> Eddowes' syndrome
> Gram's stain
> Homans' test
> Osgood-Schlatter disease
> Richards clamp
> *but:*
> The Billroth operation was successful.
> A Brudzinski reflex was elicited.
> A Gram stain showed . . .

For eponymic names of surgical instruments, do **not** use the possessive form.

Allis forceps	Hegar dilators	Jackson retractor
Tessier elevators	Yasargil knife	Watts tenaculum
Kevorkian curet	Gigli saw	Freer elevator
Jones tube	Sarns saw	Sims retractor

Possessive compound nouns: For plural compound nouns containing a possessive, use the singular possessive form for the first noun and make the second noun plural.

> bachelor's degrees   master's degrees   driver's licenses

Possessive phrases or name combinations: For phrases or name combinations, show possession in the last word only.

> Diehl and Fordney's text
> Miller and Keane's book
> Sloane and Dusseau's new pathology word book
> the chief of staff's announcement
> the Governor of Maine's statement

When possession is common to two or more individuals, show possession in the last name only. If possession is not common, show possession in each name.

> Drs. Osgood and Schlatter's theory
> Tessier's and Pitman's conclusions differed.
> Bartholin's, urethral, and Skene's glands

Plurals of single letters, symbols, and lowercase abbreviations: Use an apostrophe to form the plural of single letters, symbols, and abbreviations written in the lowercase.

+'s
serial K's ranged from . . .
wbc's (*but* WBCs if uppercase is used)

Plurals of all-capital abbreviations: It is preferred to form the plural of all-capital abbreviations without the use of an apostrophe.

EOMs are full.   rare PVCs   serial EKGs

Plurals of brief forms: For abbreviations which are brief forms of the full word, form the plural by adding **s** without an apostrophe.

bands   lymphs   segs   polys   exams

Plurals of numbers: Do not use an apostrophe to form the plural of numbers.

blood sugars in the low 100s

Plurals of abbreviated units of measure: For abbreviated units of measure, the singular and plural forms are the same; do not add apostrophe or **s** to form the plural.

5 mg   3 cc   8 lb.   10 cm   4 h.

Plurals of names: Do not use an apostrophe to form the plural of a name.

Babinskis were negative.
The master patient index lists hundreds of Joneses.

CAPITALIZATION

Beginning of sentence: Capitalize the first letter of each sentence.

Aspirin failed to relieve the pain.

Insert the word "the" to avoid beginning a sentence with certain words that should never be capitalized.

Right: The pH was 7.43.

Wrong: PH was 7.43.
Wrong: pH was 7.43.

Headings: Capitalize major headings in medical reports. Underline and/or follow the heading with a colon, depending on the style of the institution. Sample major headings for the basic reports are indicated below. Individual reports may have variable wording, deletions, or additions.

HISTORY AND PHYSICAL EXAMINATION

CHIEF COMPLAINT
HISTORY OF PRESENT ILLNESS
PAST HISTORY
SOCIAL HISTORY
FAMILY HISTORY
REVIEW OF SYSTEMS
PHYSICAL EXAMINATION
ADMITTING DIAGNOSIS (or IMPRESSION)
PLAN

CONSULTATION

Similar to above, plus
DATA BASE
ASSESSMENT
RECOMMENDATIONS

DISCHARGE SUMMARY

ADMITTING DIAGNOSIS
HISTORY OF PRESENT ILLNESS
PERTINENT PAST HISTORY
LABORATORY FINDINGS
HOSPITAL COURSE
DISPOSITION
FOLLOWUP
CONDITION ON DISCHARGE
DISCHARGE DIAGNOSES (or FINAL DIAGNOSES)
PROGNOSIS
DISCHARGE MEDICATIONS

OPERATIVE REPORT

PREOPERATIVE DIAGNOSIS
POSTOPERATIVE DIAGNOSIS
ANESTHESIA
FINDINGS
PROCEDURE

PROBLEM-ORIENTED MEDICAL RECORD

SUBJECTIVE
OBJECTIVE
ASSESSMENT
PLAN

Allergies: Some institutions use all capitals to identify allergies in medical reports.

ALLERGIES: PENICILLIN AND ASPIRIN.

Series: In series listed vertically, capitalize the first letter of each entry (numbered or not); lowercase other words unless they are always capitalized. Use of a period at the end of each entry demonstrates it is complete.

FINAL DIAGNOSES:
Severe arthritis.
Anxiety depression.
Advanced Parkinson's disease.

ADMITTING DIAGNOSIS:
1. Chest pain, suspect angina.
2. Pulmonary emphysema.
3. Family history of Crohn's disease.

In a series written horizontally in paragraph form, use uppercase for the first word of a full sentence following the colon; use lowercase if an incomplete sentence follows the colon. (See also next section, **Following a colon.**)

Reasons for referral: The patient has end-stage renal disease. He also has complications of brittle diabetes mellitus including diabetic retinitis and nonhealing foot ulcers.

The patient's medical history includes the following: chronic silicosis, status post left thoracotomy for removal of multiple cocci nodules, arteriosclerotic cardiovascular disease, and mild chronic seizure disorder.

Following a colon: After a colon, capitalize the first word when two or more clipped sentences follow. For additional examples, see the section on **Grammar,** pp. 26-27.

Heart: Regular rhythm. No murmurs heard.

Lowercase items in a series following a colon.

The patient had a history of multiple diagnoses, including the following: chronic silicosis, status post left thoracotomy for removal of multiple cocci nodules, arteriosclerotic cardiovascular disease, mild chronic seizure disorder.

NOTE: In the physical examination, where some subheadings may be followed by colons and clipped sentences or phrases and some may not, be consistent in style. Capitalize the first word after each colon.

Chest: No rales or rhonchi.   Heart: Regular rhythm.   Abdomen: Soft. Normal bowel sounds. No organomegaly.

Greek letters: Do not capitalize the English translations of Greek letters.

alpha   beta   delta   gamma

Official names: Capitalize official names of institutions and their departments. Lowercase non-official references to them.

>Mercy Hospital
>Mercy Hospital Emergency Room
>Department of Surgery, Mercy Hospital
>Board of Trustees, Mercy Hospital
>Department of Pathology, Mercy Hospital
>Orthopedic Clinic, Mercy Hospital
>Social Service Department, Mercy Hospital
>the board of trustees
>the surgical department
>the emergency room
>the operating room
>the orthopedic clinic
>a pathology report
>a pediatric consultation
>a social service consult
>the recovery room
>the vascular surgery team

Medical specialties: Do not capitalize the names of medical or surgical specialties or the physicians designated as specialists in those areas.

>evaluation from an orthopedist
>a rehabilitation consultant suggested
>the consultant's findings

Races and ethnic groups: Capitalize the names of races and ethnic groups, but do not capitalize designations based on skin color.

black	white
Negro	Caucasian
Indian	Eurasian
Oriental	Hispanic

Categories and classifications: It is preferable to lowercase terms which categorize or classify.

class	class IV Pap smear
grade	grade 1/6 systolic murmur
grade	cancer grades 1–4
lead	EKG leads V1 and V2
series	gastrointestinal series (GI series)
stage	cancer stages I–IV
type	type IIb hyperlipoproteinemia

Gravida, para, ab: While it is acceptable to capitalize the following words, the preferred form is with lowercase letters.

>gravida   para   ab

Anatomic features: Do not capitalize the Latin or English names of anatomic features. Capitalize eponyms associated with anatomic features.

arteria perinealis
ligament of Treitz
musculus auricularis anterior
nervus mentalis
os frontale
renal artery
space of Retzius
temporal bone
venae ciliares

Genus and species names: Capitalize the singular form of the name of a genus, whether accompanied or not by the species name. Do not capitalize the species name.

Aspergillus	Aspergillus auricularis
Campylobacter	Campylobacter jejuni
Diplococcus	Diplococcus pneumoniae
Escherichia	Escherichia coli
Hemophilus	Hemophilus influenzae
Mycoplasma	Mycoplasma hominis
Staphylococcus	Staphylococcus aureus
Streptococcus	Streptococcus pneumoniae
Trichomonas	Trichomonas vaginalis

Capitalize the single-letter abbreviation of a genus name, but do not use the abbreviation unless it is accompanied by the species name and it has previously been expressed in full in the same report. Use a period following the abbreviation. Do not capitalize or abbreviate the species name.

E. coli   H. influenzae

Do not capitalize the plural or adjectival form of a genus name.

Singular	Plural	Adjective
Aspergillus	aspergilli	
Diplococcus	diplococci	diplococcal
Mycoplasma	mycoplasmas	mycoplasmal
	mycoplasmata	
Staphylococcus	staphylococci	staphylococcal
Streptococcus	streptococci	streptococcal
Trichomonas		trichomonal

Virus names: Lowercase most virus names. Consult references for guidance. Capitalize alphabetical designations.

herpesvirus
group B coxsackievirus

Trade or brand names: Capitalize trade names or brand names of drugs, sutures, instruments, etc. Do not capitalize generic names, chemical names, or descriptive terms.

Alupent	imipramine
Bacitracin ointment	milk of magnesia
bronchodilators	nylon sutures
Bronkometer	Randall forceps
codeine	ring forceps
Dexon sutures	Valium
erythromycin	Vicryl sutures
Ethiflex sutures	Zyloprim

Lowercase drug names which may be either generic or brand, unless it is certain that the brand drug is being referred to.

He responded well to aminophylline (*not* Aminophyllin).

Reference books on medications differ internally and among themselves in their presentations of brand names, e.g., initial capital only, all capital, a mix of capital and lowercase letters. Even a manufacturer's packaging and promotional or descriptive material on a drug may have variations. It is acceptable to use only an initial capital when the definitive presentation cannot be determined.

HydroDIURIL, Hydrodiuril, HydroDiuril
pHisoHex, Phisohex
RhoGAM, RhoGam, Rhogam
Nitro-Bid, Nitro-bid
SER-AP-ES, Ser-Ap-Es, Ser-ap-es
Theo-Dur, Theo-dur
Gore-Tex, Gore-tex
E.E.S., EES

Do not capitalize a common noun following a trade or brand name.

Nitro-Bid capsules   Adaptic dressing   Mylanta tablets   Kay Ciel elixir

Do not capitalize adjectives associated with trade or brand names.

intravenous Valium   running Dacron sutures

Eponyms: Capitalize the eponymic names of operations, procedures, instruments, incisions, anatomic features, etc.   Consult references to determine which names are eponymic. Do not capitalize the noun an eponym is combined with.

Auer rods	Crohn's disease	Ellik evacuator
Graves' disease	Homans' test	Jackson-Pratt drain
ligament of Treitz	Pfannenstiel incision	space of Retzius

Capitalize eponyms but do not capitalize words derived from eponymic names.

Gram's stain   *but:* gram-positive cocci, gram-negative stain

Cushing's syndrome	*but:*	cushingoid facies
Parkinson's disease	*but:*	parkinsonian syndrome
Jackson's syndrome	*but:*	jacksonian seizures or epilepsy

Small bleeders were coagulated with Bovie cautery.
but:
Small bleeders were bovied.

The patient underwent cesarean section.

Do not capitalize adjectives associated with eponymic names.

red Robinson catheter

Abbreviations: Capitalize most abbreviations which are formed from selected letters of the phrase abbreviated. Do not use periods.

BUN	blood urea nitrogen
CBC	complete blood count
CABG	coronary artery bypass graft
URI	upper respiratory infection

Capitalize abbreviations composed of letters from a single word. Do not use periods.

GU	genitourinary
GI	gastrointestinal series
IV	intravenous
IM	intramuscular

Acronyms: Capitalize all the letters of an acronym (composed of initial letters of successive words in a phrase, and pronounced as a word). Do not use periods.

FANA   PERRLA   TED   MAST   TORCH

Do not capitalize acronyms which have become words themselves.

laser   fabere   rem   dopa

Brief forms: Do not capitalize brief forms of words and do not use a period following the brief form.

ab   exam   lab   sed rate   prep   flu

Chemical symbols: Lowercase chemical elements and compounds when they are written in full. Capitalize the initial letter of the abbreviation of each chemical element.

oxygen	O_2
iron	Fe (initial capital only)
ferrous sulfate	$FeSO_4$

pO2 and pCO2:   The abbreviations for partial pressure of oxygen and partial pressure of carbon dioxide may be written as either pO2 and pCO2, or PO2 and PCO2. Medical references which capitalize the **P** use a different size capital than that used for the chemical symbols O2 or CO2. Since this is not possible on standard keyboards, the lowercase **p** is preferred to better differentiate it from the chemical symbol **P** for phosphorus. Do not use periods. Do not place a hyphen between the **O** and the **2.**

> Preferred: pO2   pCO2
> Acceptable: PO2   PCO2

pH: The only correct way to write **pH** is to lowercase the **p,** uppercase the **H.** Do not space between the letters; do not use periods. If a sentence starts with the abbreviation **pH,** insert the word "The" before it.

> The pH was 4.5.

Units of measure: Lowercase units of measure. Abbreviations of units of measure are generally lowercase, except for some units of measure derived from proper names. Consult references for guidance.

decibel	dB or db	gram	g or gm
meter	m	watt	W
kilogram	kg	hertz	Hz

COLONS

Enumeration: Use a colon before an enumeration, including findings related to subheadings, e.g., in the review of systems or physical examination. Often a colon follows a phrase such as "the following" or "as follows." Do not substitute a hyphen (-) or dash (—) for a colon.

> Medications: Theo-Dur, prednisone, Bronkometer.

> HEENT: Much dental work is noted. Teeth in fair repair. EOMs full. PERRLA. Fundi benign. Neck is supple, nontender.

> The patient had multiple diagnoses including the following: chronic silicosis, status post left thoracotomy for removal of multiple cocci nodules, and mild chronic seizure disorder.

If the content follows on the same line as a major heading in a medical report, use a colon following the heading.

> ADMISSION DIAGNOSES: Gastroenteritis.
>   Dehydration.

The colon is optional if the heading stands alone on a line and the content begins on a separate line.

ADMISSION DIAGNOSES
Gastroenteritis.
Dehydration.

or

ADMISSION DIAGNOSES:
Gastroenteritis.
Dehydration.

Do not use a colon if the enumeration follows a verb.

Medications taken are Theo-Dur, prednisone, Bronkometer.
Abdomen is soft, nontender, without masses or organomegaly.

Time and equator or meridian readings: Use a colon to express time when hours and minutes are given, and to express equator or meridian readings. Exception: Do not use a colon in military or 24-hour time, e.g., 1830 hours (6:30 p.m.).

8:30 a.m., 0830 hours

11:40 p.m., 2340 hours

sclerotomy drainage at 8:30 equator

Ratios: Express ratios with arabic numerals and the colon sign (:). No space precedes or follows the colon.

Mycoplasma 1:2 *(Dictated:* "Mycoplasma one to two")

cold agglutinins 1:4 *(Dictated:* " . . . one to four")

Zolyse 1:10,000 *(Dictated:* ". . . one to ten thousand")

NOTE: A **range** may be dictated the same way as a ratio but is written differently. A range is expressed with the word "to" or a hyphen, not a colon.

blood sugars in the range of 80 to 125 . . .
blood sugars in the range of 80–125 . . .

Heart disease: When giving the etiologic, anatomic, and physiologic diagnosis of heart disease, use a colon following each heading. The functional class may or may not be preceded by a title, e.g., cardiac class or prognosis.

Heart disease cannot be ruled out. Etiology: Arteriosclerotic. Anatomic: Coronary artery disease. Physiologic: EKG shows poor R-wave progression in V1 through V3, consistent with an old transmural infarction of the anteroseptal myocardium. Functional class 2.

COMMAS

Independent clauses: Use a comma to separate two independent clauses joined by **and, but, for, or, nor, yet,** or **so.** (The comma is optional if the two sentences are short and their meanings will not be confused.)

> There is no constipation, but there are skin changes and cold intolerance noted.

> A venogram was positive for deep vein thrombosis, and he was placed on bedrest and heparin.

> Breath sounds were distant, and rhonchi were appreciated throughout.
> *or*
> Breath sounds were distant and rhonchi were appreciated throughout.

NOTE: Do not use a comma before **and, but, for, or, nor, yet,** or **so** if it is followed by a phrase or a second verb without a new subject.

> The patient presented without acute problems but with a long history of tiredness and depression.

> The patient had nausea but had not vomited with the present illness.

Series: Use a comma to separate items in a simple series. When the items in a series number three or more, a final comma before **and, or,** or **nor** is optional unless its presence or absence influences the meaning. Use a semicolon to separate items in a complex series. (See section titled **Semicolons.)**

> **Final comma optional:**

> Ears, nose, and throat are normal.
> Ears, nose and throat are normal.

> **Final comma required:**

> No dysphagia, hoarseness, or enlargement of the thyroid gland.
> (Omission of the final comma would incorrectly join hoarseness, as well as enlargement, with "of the thyroid gland.")

> **Final comma must not be used:**

> Hemoglobin of 14.8, hematocrit 44.6, WBC 14,000 with 71 segs and 21 lymphs (*or* 71% segs and 21% lymphs). (The segs and lymphs together describe the differential of the white blood count.)

> Blood sugar initially was 46 mg%, creatinine and BUN normal.
> (Both creatinine and BUN were normal.)

For clarity: Use a comma to enhance clarity and to avoid confusion.

> The patient will be sent home on 18 units of NPH and 8 units of regular in the morning, and 6 units of regular and 6 units of NPH insulin before supper.

> The patient made an uneventful recovery and was discharged without medicines other than his premorbid medicines, to be treated at home and followed in the office.

Opening adverbial phrases or clauses: While a comma following an opening adverbial phrase or clause is optional, the trend is to omit it unless its absence causes confusion. When there is a single introductory word, omit the comma.

> **Comma optional:**
>
> While in the hospital a CAT scan was done.
> While in the hospital, a CAT scan was done.
>
> Associated with this he had numbness of the left face.
> Associated with this, he had numbness of the left face.
>
> With regard to the patient's stamina she feels that she has no excessive shortness of breath.
> With regard to the patient's stamina, she feels that she has no excessive shortness of breath.
>
> Although she sleeps fairly well she feels tired on awakening.
> Although she sleeps fairly well, she feels tired on awakening.
>
> At that time she had developed PVCs intermittently.
> At that time, she had developed PVCs intermittently.

> **Omit the comma:**
> Presently she takes no medications for this particular problem.

> **Comma required for clarity:**
> Because of vomiting, an NG tube was put in place.

Adjectives: Use commas to separate two or more adjectives if each modifies the noun alone. Do not place a comma between the last adjective and the noun the series modifies.

> Physical exam reveals a pleasant, cooperative, elderly female in no acute distress.
> The abdomen is soft, nontender.

If an adjective modifies a combination of the following adjective(s) and noun, do not use a comma to separate the adjectives.

> He had a traumatic neck fracture.
> This 54-year-old Caucasian female was referred to our office for evaluation.
> She did not present with audible paroxysmal tachycardia.

Use commas to set off an adjective or adjectival clause directly following the noun it modifies.

> Pain is greatly increased in both knees, left greater than right.

. . . degenerative arthritis, left knee, with increasing inability to cope . . .

Blood cultures were drawn at different times, all of which were negative.

Nonessential words or phrases: Use commas to set off nonessential subordinate or participial words or phrases which interrupt the flow of the sentence. The use of commas to set off other nonessential words or phrases is optional and the trend is to avoid using them.

Comma required:

Blood cultures were drawn at different times, all of which were negative.
Serum vitamin B12 level was 598, well within the normal limits.
Ultimately this cleared, however, and azotemia too was reversed.
Physical on admission, other than revealing pallor and weakness, was within normal limits.
There was diffuse tenderness throughout, more pronounced in the lower abdomen.
The reason for admission was to, as already stated, begin therapy with an insulin pump.
During her hospital stay, because of the auricular fibrillation being the possible source of vascular aneurysm of the central nervous system, it was elected to start her on anti-coagulant therapy.

Comma optional:

. . . white count 8600, with a normal differential
X-ray showed an ulnar styloid process fracture, for which the patient was wearing a cast on admission.
Unfortunately the patient continued to smoke, although he was chastised for this.
He was seen in consultation by Dr. Jones, who did an upper tract endoscopy.
Deep tendon reflexes $2+/4+$, with brisk return phase.
We also did a colonoscopy, looking for a right colonic lesion, which was fortunately not found. (First comma preferred, second optional.)

Essential phrases: Do not use commas to set off essential phrases.

This 77-year-old housewife entered with acute faintness and rapid heart action.
Ticarcillin was continued up to the present time because of his marked granulocytopenia.
The patient is a 43-year-old Caucasian male who was admitted to the hospital on the evening of the 25th with an abnormal blood count having been discovered that day.
This 54-year-old Caucasian female is presenting without acute problems but with a long history of tiredness and depression.
The left breast shows a large depression in the superior-lateral quadrant where previous surgery had been performed.

Transitional phrases: When a transitional phrase of independent comment occurs at the beginning of a second independent clause and it is preceded by a comma and **and, but, for, or, nor, yet,** or **so,** follow the transitional phrase with a comma.

He was much less encephalopathic, but despite the infusions of half-normal saline, he still betrayed the presence of orthostatic hypotension.

Drug dosage and instructions: To reduce clutter and increase clarity, it is recommended that commas not be used to separate drug names from dosage and instructions. In a series of drugs for each of which the dosage and/or instructions are given, use a comma (or semicolon) to separate each complete entry. The semicolon is preferred if entries in the series have internal commas.

The patient was discharged on Coumadin 10 mg daily.

The patient was discharged on the following regimen: theophylline 15 cc four times a day; Carafate 1 gm four times a day, 30 minutes after meals and one at bedtime; bethanechol 25 mg p.o. q.i.d.; and Reglan 5 mg at bedtime on a trial basis.

He was finally sent home on erythromycin 500 mg q.i.d., Theo-Dur 300 mg b.i.d., and Tenormin 50 mg q.d.
or
He was finally sent home on erythromycin 500 mg q.i.d.; Theo-Dur 300 mg b.i.d.; and Tenormin 50 mg q.d.

Laboratory values: To reduce clutter and increase clarity, it is recommended that commas not be used to separate a lab value from the test it describes. When multiple lab results are reported, separate related tests by commas, unrelated tests by periods.

LABORATORY EXAMINATION: Sodium 139, potassium 4.6, chloride 106, bicarb 28, BUN 15, creatinine 0.9. White count 5.9, hemoglobin 14.6, hematocrit 43.1. PT 11.3, PTT 31.4. Urinalysis: pH 6, specific gravity 1.006, negative dipstick and negative microscopic exam. Chest x-ray revealed no acute disease. EKG: Normal sinus rhythm, rate 68, PR 0.20, QRS 0.08, QT 0.42, axis +60°.

Dates: Place a comma before and after the year if it is preceded by the day of the month and the sentence continues beyond it.

The patient was admitted on December 14, 1983, and discharged on January 4, 1984.

Commas omitted:
The patient's previous admissions were in March 1982 and June 1983.
The patient was admitted on 14 December 1983 and discharged on 4 January 1984.

Geography: Place commas before and after the state name preceded by a city name, or a country name preceded by a state or city name.

The patient is from Marshall, Texas, and moved to Modesto, California, 15 years ago.

The patient recently traveled to New South Wales, Australia, and Auckland, New Zealand.

Since the patient's return from vacation in Penzance, Cornwall, England, she has suffered from excessive weight loss, fatigue, and insomnia.

Quantities: Use a comma to indicate thousands. The comma may be omitted in numbers ranging from 1000 to 9999.

Platelet count was 353,000.
White count was 7,100.
White count was 7100.

Latin abbreviations: Place a comma before and after Latin abbreviations used parenthetically within a sentence.

etc.   and so forth
e.g.   for example
i.e.   that is
et al.   and others

The functional class may be preceded by a title, e.g., cardiac class or prognosis.

EDITING

Definition:

Editing in the medical record can range from a simple grammatical change, such as correcting plural or singular or punctuation, to correcting a medical inconsistency or deleting an inappropriate remark by a physician. In between, there are decisions to be made ranging from educated analysis to second guessing what the physician is trying to say and saying it better, to leaving a blank altogether.

How each editing situation is handled can depend on many factors: experience in a similar situation, knowledge of the physician's dictating habits, experience in the field, type of transcription setting, amount of physician contact. . . .

(Kathy Bennett, "An Introduction to Editing," in "Editing Practices in Medical Transcription," *Journal of the American Association for Medical Transcription,* Vol. 1, No. 1, Summer 1982, p. 38.)

How and when to edit:

In editing dictation, we do not go charging in, doctoring up the reports in an aggressive way, in an intrusional way. It has to be done so subtly, so delicately, so carefully, that we get a favorable response from the dictator.

. . .

We must be so involved with what we are transcribing that we know what is going on and can detect something that is dictated that does not make sense, that does not flow, that does not add up. We must listen with an educated ear, with an intelligent ear, so that we can produce an accurate, intelligent, clear document, always remembering the fine line between **editing** *and* **tampering.**

(Vera Pyle, "The Editing Function of the Medical Transcriptionist," in "Editing Practices in Medical Transcription," *Journal of the American Association for Medical Transcription,* Vol. 1, No. 1, Summer 1982, p. 42.)

When not to edit:

What about those who are inconsiderate of us? What about those who mumble? What about those whom we can't help because we don't know what they mean? If you know what they are trying to say, you can help clarify the dictation. If you don't know, that is the time to transcribe verbatim; it's our only recourse (Pyle, p. 42).

Guidelines: Throughout transcription, it is important to retain the dictating physician's style. It is not our place to impose our style on the report; it is our responsibility to produce clear, accurate, and complete reports.

Hospital or department policy and physician preference are major factors in decisions to edit. To the extent that editing is acceptable in your setting and to the dictating physician, the following guidelines for editing are recommended.

Edit grammatical, punctuation, spelling, and similar dictation errors as necessary to achieve clear communication. See sections addressing these areas for additional guidelines and examples.

Edit slang words and phrases, incorrect or verbal inconsistencies, and medical inconsistencies.

Dictated:	FEV/FVC **ratio** is 38%.
Transcribed:	FEV/FVC **value** is 38% (*or* FEV/FVC is 38%.)

Dictated:	The patient has had persistent enlarged liver for some time and has been on medications for this purpose.
Transcribed:	The patient has had persistent enlarged liver for some time and has been on medications for this.
	(The medication was to treat the enlarged liver, not to cause it or increase it.)

Dictated:	The morning after the dex . . .
Transcribed:	The morning after the dexamethasone . . .

Dictated:	temp spike
Transcribed:	temperature spike

Edit inaccurate phrasing of laboratory data.

Dictated:	Hemoglobin was "seven two."
Transcribed:	Hemoglobin was 7.2.

Dictated:	specific gravity "ten thirty"
Transcribed:	specific gravity 1.030

Dictated:	blood sugars in the "2 to 3 hundred range"
Transcribed:	blood sugars in the 200 to 300 range

Normal/negative findings: Never delete negative or normal findings as dictated by the physician. To do so is tampering with the dictation as well as with the medical record. In medical care, normal or negative findings may be as significant, unique, and pertinent as abnormal or positive findings. Recording them may limit unnecessary repetition of tests or procedures to determine findings, thus reducing the cost of health care. It is not the transcriptionist's place to judge or exclude normal/negative findings when they are dictated.

Procedure for correcting errors in dictation: Use the patient's medical record to clarify or correct dictation. If the record is not available, draw attention to errors or potentially confusing entries for which you do not have sufficient information to make corrections.

Leave a blank space in a report rather than guessing what was meant or transcribing unclear or obviously incorrect dictation. Flag the report to draw attention to the blank and seek the correct information.

> Dictated: The temperature at the time of discharge was **57.4.**
> Transcribed: The temperature at the time of discharge was ＿＿.

Attach a note indicating that "57.4" was dictated and the chart was not available to determine whether 37.4 C or 97.4 F (or some other value) was correct.

When flagging a report to draw attention to unclear or incorrect dictation, cite the page, section, and line number; place a faint pencil mark in the margin to assist in locating the problem area. If the word or phrase is unfamiliar, note what it sounds like. If the term is inconsistent, briefly state why, e.g., "Patient initially described as having a **left** below-knee amputation, later referred to as **right** BK amputation. Which is correct?"

Similarly, draw attention to major medical inconsistencies you have corrected, in order to permit physician review to assure accuracy.

When transcribing dictation by physicians who speak English as a second language, edit obvious errors, following the general guidelines for editing. It is not necessary or recommended that such dictation be rewritten; rather, the physician's basic style should be retained.

Edit inappropriate language or inflammatory remarks, such as the following:

> Dictated: The red inflamed cervix against the background of the patient's bright green dress was reminiscent of a South American parrot.
> Transcribed: The cervix was red and inflamed.

Medical record/transcription office settings should provide written instructions to deal with these and other types of inappropriate remarks. Medical transcriptionists should check with the supervisors of their own facilities to determine the rules for editing or omitting inappropriate remarks from the transcription. The following examples are quoted from Kathy Bennett, "An Introduction to Editing," in "Editing Practices in Medical Transcription," *Journal of the American Association for Medical Transcription,* Vol. 1, No. 1, Summer 1982, p. 39.

> *The cervix looked like it had been through World War II.*

> *The patient was treated with substandard medical care due to the fact that a typed cardiac catheterization was not on the chart at the time of treatment, and a handwritten report was totally illegible and worthless in the treatment of the patient.*

FORMAT

Headings: Title sections of reports as dictated. Use all capitals for major headings. Underlining is optional.

For admitting diagnoses, impressions, discharge diagnoses, preoperative diagnoses, postoperative diagnoses, names of operations, and similar headings, list vertically the entries which follow. Numbering should be used if dictated; it is optional if not. If the physician numbers some but not all items in a series, number all or none of the entries when transcribing.

Entries following major headings may begin either on the same line or on the following line:

DIAGNOSES: Severe arthritis.
　　　　　　　Anxiety depression.

DIAGNOSES:
1. Fatty necrosis of the liver, secondary to ethanol consumption, but rule out carcinoma metastases.
2. Hypertensive cardiovascular disease, under control.
3. Hepatic failure, cirrhosis of the liver.

HOSPITAL COURSE: Chest x-ray was obtained in the emergency room . . .

HOSPITAL COURSE:
Chest x-ray was obtained in the emergency room . . .

Subheadings: Subheadings of report sections may be listed vertically or horizontally. Likewise, they may be capitalized or not in either format.

Head:　　　Normocephalic.
Eyes:　　　PERRLA. EOMs full.
Neck:　　　Supple.
Chest:　　　Clear to percussion and auscultation.
Abdomen:　Soft, nontender.

HEAD: Normocephalic. EYES: PERRLA. EOMs full. NECK: Supple.
CHEST: Clear to percussion and auscultation. ABDOMEN: Soft, nontender.

Obvious headings which are not dictated may be inserted, but this is not required.

Dictated:　　The patient's family history is noncontributory.
Transcribed:　As dictated, or
　　　　　　　FAMILY HISTORY: Noncontributory.

If the physician does not dictate complete sections but moves in and out of sections, it may be preferable to omit headings.

Standard format: While various institutional formats are acceptable, it is recommended that the general format of the basic four reports (histories and physicals, consultations, operative reports, and discharge summaries) be consistent within an institution.

It is further recommended that a single standard form be used for all of the basic four reports, including continuation sheets. Except for sections for institutional and patient identification data, no paragraph or section headings should be preprinted on the forms.

Utilization of standard forms without preprinted headings permits the physician's dictating style to determine the sequence and length of entries, improves productivity of the medical transcriptionist, and reduces costs of supplies and production.

Continuation sheets: When a medical report is longer than one page, the patient's name, medical record number, and the page number should be typed on each continuation sheet. Additional data may be noted, depending on the institution's preference.

The continuation sheets may be headed in the vertical flush-left format or the horizontal format.

```
David Bryon
#584681
Page 2
```

or:

David Bryon   #584681   Page 2

Do not carry a single line of a report onto a continuation sheet. Do not place only the signature block on a continuation sheet.

Signature line: Space four to six lines between the end of the report and the signature line.

GRAMMAR

Clipped sentences: While complete sentences are the grammatically correct form, it is often the physician's style to dictate in clipped sentences. This is acceptable in medical reports because it provides direct, succinct content, at the same time reflecting the physician's style.

It is not unusual for the laboratory data, review of systems, and physical examination to be dictated in clipped sentences, while complete sentences are used in the remaining sections (history and hospital course). Such a mix is acceptable.

The physician's preference may determine whether clipped sentences are to be transcribed as dictated or should be expanded into complete sentences. If the usual style is to dictate in clipped sentences, it is recommended not to expand these into complete sentences unless it is known that the physician prefers this. An occasional clipped sentence within a narrative section of a report (history, hospital course) is easily expanded into a complete sentence and makes the section internally consistent.

When transcribing clipped sentences, follow general punctuation rules within them. Do not clip sentences unless they are so dictated.

HEENT: Normocephalic. Teeth in poor repair. Fundi benign.

Blood pressure 134/70, pulse 100, respirations 18.

Followup in my office in approximately a week.

A 36-year-old white female admitted after experiencing cough and fever x 2 weeks. Seen in office, with chest x-ray revealing right upper lobe pneumonia. Admitted for control of symptoms, further evaluation, and pulmonary consult.

Mycoplasma 1:8. White count 7,000. Hemoglobin and hematocrit 13.1 and 39.

SOCIAL HISTORY: Smokes. Uses alcohol. Has three children.

Dictated: A 79-year-old white male with a long history of known diagnoses. He has a history of daily cough. He was followed as an outpatient. However, he did not improve substantially. He was admitted . . .

May be transcribed as dictated or: This is a 79-year-old white male with a long history of known diagnoses. He has a history . . .

Noun-verb agreement in number: Use a singular verb with a singular subject, a plural verb with a plural subject. Correct any dictation which mixes the two.

Dictated:	Medications taken **is** Tylenol and Flexeril.
Transcribed:	Medications taken **are** Tylenol and Flexeril.

Dictated:	The patient brought in some fish sticks which she felt **was** the cause of her infection.
Transcribed:	The patient brought in some fish sticks which she felt **were** the cause of her infection.

Dictated:	There **has** been no recent injuries.
Transcribed:	There **have** been no recent injuries.

Dictated:	Marked diverticulosis and diverticulitis **was** noted.
Transcribed:	Marked diverticulosis and diverticulitis **were** noted.

If the subject consists of one or more singular words connected by **or** or **nor,** or the conjunctions **either...or, neither...nor, not only...but also,** the verb is singular.

No bruit or venous hum is noted.

If the subject consists of one or more plural words connected by **or** or **nor,** or the conjunctions **either...or, neither...nor, not only...but also,** the verb is plural.

> No bruits or venous hums are noted.

If the subject consists of singular and plural words connected by **or** or **nor,** or the conjunctions **either...or, neither...nor, not only...but also,** the verb agrees with the number of the nearer subject.

Dictated:	There **were** no organomegaly or masses.
Transcribed:	There **was** no organomegaly or masses.

Dictated:	No masses or discharge **are** present.
Transcribed:	No masses or discharge **is** present.

Always use a singular verb with units of measure.

Dictated:	Twenty milliequivalents of KCl **were** given.
Transcribed:	Twenty milliequivalents of KCl **was** given.

Tense: Physicians often switch tenses within a report. The transcriptionist should try to be consistent, typing the report either in the present or past tense.

General rules: A history is past tense and a physical exam is usually in the present tense, but past tense is acceptable. Consultation reports: Past tense for history and previous findings, present or past tense for physical examination, present tense for recommendations. Operations: Past tense, unless physician dictates as he or she operates. Discharge summary: Past tense except for discharge instructions and plan.

Awkwardness: Improve awkward phrasing in dictation:

Dictated:	Breasts: Large pendulous breasts **being** present. No masses or discharge is noted.
Transcribed:	Breasts: Large pendulous breasts **are** present. No masses or discharge is noted.

Dictated:	. . . increasing inability **with** coping with usual functional daily demands of living.
Transcribed:	. . . increasing inability **to** cope with . . .

Articles *a* and *an:* Use **an** before words beginning with a vowel sound; use **a** before words beginning with a consonant sound.

Dictated:	. . . **a** allergic cutaneous reaction
Transcribed:	. . . **an** allergic cutaneous reaction

Dictated:	**a** old chorioretinal scar
Transcribed:	**an** old chorioretinal scar

HYPHENS

Hyphens may be used to divide words at the ends of lines. However, in transcribing medical reports, the avoidance of such word division is preferred. This elimination of word division enhances communication and production: unhyphenated words are easier to read and faster to type since the transcriptionist need not take time to determine correct word division.

See the section titled **Word Division** (pp. 35-36) for general rules on end-of-line word division.

Avoid using hyphens at the end of more than two consecutive lines.

Do not end a page with a hyphen.

Compound adjectives: Use hyphens to connect most compound adjectives (multiple-word modifiers) which precede a noun. Omit the hyphens if the compound adjective follows the noun.

This 54-year-old woman was referred for evaluation.
but: The woman referred for evaluation is 54 years old.

NOTE: If fractions are used in the age, hyphenate as in the following examples.

This 7-1/2-year-old girl . . .
This 7½-year-old girl . . .
This girl is 7-1/2 years old.
This girl is 7½ years old.

This is a well-nourished, well-developed patient.
but: The patient is well nourished and well developed.

Sputum showed many gram-positive rods.
but: Sputum showed rods which were gram positive.

He has biopsy-proven silicosis.
but: His silicosis is biopsy proven.

Sonography showed an ill-defined mass.
but: The mass on sonography was ill defined.

before-breakfast blood sugars
but: Blood sugars will be drawn before breakfast.

He had a low-grade temperature.
but: His temperature was low grade.

well-encapsulated mass
but: The mass was well encapsulated.

Roux-en-Y operation
self-retaining retractor

to-and-fro murmur
small-volume nebulizer
zero-release aspirin
nasal-prong O2
end-to-side anastomosis
left-to-right shunt
cul-de-sac
24-hour free cortisol
fast-food restaurant
iron-binding capacity
five-pound weight gain
low-grade fever
high-dose intravenous penicillin
low-dose heparin
gram-positive cocci
full-blown history of severe bleeding
Twenty-four hours after admission . . .

Disease-entity modifiers: Do not use a hyphen with disease-entity modifiers.

arteriosclerotic cardiovascular disease
cervical disk disease
congestive heart failure
oat cell carcinoma
organic brain syndrome
pelvic inflammatory disease
rheumatic heart disease
sickle cell disease
upper respiratory tract infection
urinary tract infection

Words as a unit: Some words are so commonly used together that they are read as a unit. Do not join these with hyphens.

arterial blood gases
blood pressure readings
deep tendon reflexes
exercise tolerance test
jugular venous distention
left lower quadrant, left upper lobe
low back pain
mean cell volume
normal sinus rhythm
pulmonary function tests
red cell count
right lower lobe, right upper quadrant
status post cellulitis
ulnar styloid process

Pairs of adjectives: Hyphenate combinations of adjectives which are equal, complementary, or contrasting:

    systolic–diastolic murmur
    inferior–posterior infarction
    tibial–calcaneal fusion

Clarity: Use the hyphen to clarify meaning.

    small-bowel obstruction (obstruction of the small bowel)
    small bowel obstruction (small obstruction of the bowel)

Eponyms: Use a hyphen to join two or more eponymic names used as multiple-word modifiers of operations, procedures, instruments, etc. Do not use a hyphen if the eponymic name refers to a single person.

    Jackson-Pratt drain
    Osgood-Schlatter disease
    but:
    Chevalier Jackson forceps (named for Dr. Chevalier Jackson)
    Austin Moore prosthesis (named for Dr. Thomas Austin Moore)

Adverbs ending in ly: Never use a hyphen after adverbs ending in **ly** when used with a participle or adjective.

    fairly chronic pain
    poorly defined mass
    slightly low albumin
    irregularly irregular rhythm
    grossly benign-appearing material
    The patient was poorly nourished.

Prefixes and suffixes: Join most common prefixes and suffixes without hyphens.

    abnormal
    afebrile, asymmetrical, asymptomatic, atraumatic
    anteroposterior, anteroseptal
    antibiotics, antibodies, antihypertensive, antitrypsin
    bigeminy, bilateral, bilobar, bimanual
    cooperative
    demineralization, desensitization
    dyspareunia
    encroachment
    epigastric
    expiratory
    extracorporeal, extraocular
    holosystolic
    hyperemesis, hyperlipoproteinemia, hyperresonant, hyperthyroid, hyperventilation
    hypoactive, hypokalemia, hypoplastic, hypotension, hypothyroid
    induction, indwelling, infiltrate, infusion, inpatient, inspiratory, intake
    intercostal, interspace

intracapsular, intracranial, intrauterine, intravenous
lightheadedness
midclavicular, midline, midlung, midback
multiview
nearsightedness
noncompliant, noncontributory, nonfasting, nonicteric, nonspecific
nontender, nonunion, nonweightbearing
onset
oropharyngeal
outlet, outpatient, output
overriding, overweight
postauricular, postbulbar, postmenopausal, postmortem
postoperative, postpartum, poststenotic
posteromedially
premedicate, premorbid, preoperative, prepatellar, presystolic
readmitted, readmission, reapproximated, rebound, reinforced
retroflexed
semicircular, semirecumbent
subperiosteally, substernal
suprapatellar, suprasternal
transmural
trilobar
ultrasound
uncomfortable, undetermined, uneventful, uninflamed, unrelieved, unremarkable

Use a hyphen when the prefix or suffix is joined with an abbreviation or number, or when it is necessary for clarity:

post–MI   post–CABG   pre–1985 admission

We will do pan–cultures.

The patient was re-appointed in one week. (The patient was given another appointment, not named again to a position. You may also recast the sentence: The patient was given an appointment in one week.)

Vowels: Use a hyphen to join word parts which, without the hyphen, would join two like vowels or result in a string of three or more vowels.

ileo–ascending colostomy
intra–abdominal
intra–articular
re–evaluate
re–examine
salpingo–oophorectomy
tubo–ovarian

Pronunciation: Use a hyphen to separate word parts when doing so makes pronunciation easier.

aorto–bifemoral bypass graft
mid–dorsum

non-interlocking, non-neoplastic
post-delivery, post-thoracentesis
pre-clotting
re-explored, re-perfusion, re-peritonealization, re-prepared, re-x-rayed

Like: Join the suffix **like** to words without the use of a hyphen unless the word is an eponym, ends in l or a vowel, or has three or more syllables.

slitlike
but:
flu-like syndrome
barrel-like chest
McBurney-like incision

Self: Use a hyphen to form **self** compounds.

self-glucose-monitoring techniques   self-assessment

Status post: Do not hyphenate the phrase **status post**; do not join **post** in this phrase to the word that follows it.

status post fractured ribs   status post cholecystectomy

Number or letter: Use a hyphen to join compound nouns which include a number or single letter.

alpha-1	alpha-2 globulin
C-section	F-wave
K-wire	profile-1
SMA-12	S-profiles
T-waves	V-plasty
x-ray	Z-incision

Chemical symbols: Never use a hyphen with chemical symbols.

O_2, *not* O-2 $FeSO_4$, *not* $FeSO-4$ or Fe-SO_4

When the mass number of a chemical element follows its symbol, use a hyphen to join the symbol and number:

I-131

Vitamins: Do not place a hyphen or space between the letter and numeral used to designate vitamins.

vitamin B1, vitamin B_1 vitamin B12, vitamin B_{12}

Optional hyphens: The following words may be hyphenated or joined without a hyphen when used as nouns or adjectives. Those which may also be used as verbs should be written separately without hyphens.

followup, follow–up, follow up (variable forms as noun, adjective, verb)
workup, work–up, work up (variable forms as noun, adjective, verb)

follow–through (noun), follow through (verb)

Noun:	I saw him in followup.
	I saw him in follow–up.
Adjective:	Followup electrocardiogram was done.
	Follow–up electrocardiogram was done.
Verb:	I will follow up his care.
Noun:	The workup was negative.
	The work–up was negative.
Adjective:	Workup results were pending.
	Work–up results were pending.
Verb:	We will work up this patient.

Series: In a series of hyphenated compounds with a common base, omit the base in all but the last. If one or more of the compounds are not hyphenated, write them in full each time.

one– to two–year history
10– to 12–second control
first– and second–degree burns
low– to moderate–voltage activity

hypothyroidism and hyperthyroidism *(not* hypo– and hyperthyroidism)

preoperative and postoperative hemoglobin *(not* pre– and postoperative hemoglobin)

midlung and lower lung fields *(not* mid and lower lung fields)

Range: In expressing a range, the words **to, through, from, between,** and **and** must be written out as follows: "from __ to __," "from __ through __," or "between __ and __." When the word **from** is not used, a hyphen may be used in place of **to** or **through.** If decimals or commas appear in the numeric values, or if values contain four or more digits, do not replace **to** or **through** with a hyphen. Do not replace **and** with an ampersand (&).

The patient's weight decreased from 52.7 kg to 51.9 kg during this hospitalization.

Hemoglobin ranged between 14.2 and 15.4 mg/dl over the course of hospitalization.

Platelet count was in the 1500 to 1600 range.

Cranial nerves II through XII were intact.
Cranial nerves II–XII were intact.

Urinalysis was negative except for 8–10 wbc.
Urinalysis was negative except for 8 to 10 wbc.

Intervertebral disk space: Use a hyphen when expressing the space between two vertebrae (the intervertebral space).

L4–L5 *or* L4–5   L5–S1   T12–L1

Suture sizes: Use a hyphen to express suture size. Alternatively, suture sizes of 1–0 through 4–0 may be expressed by the appropriate number of zeros. Avoid using more than four zeros so that the reader will not have to count zeros to determine the suture size.

3–0 nylon, or 000 nylon   *but:*   5–0 Vicryl, *not* 00000 Vicryl

Fractions: Hyphenate fractions which are written out.

one–half normal saline
two–thirds of the way up his right chest

Mixed fractions: It is preferable to use a hyphen with mixed fractions when the keyboard does not provide a single key for the fraction. The hyphen helps the reader by clearly joining the fraction with the whole number preceding it.

2–1/2   3–3/4   5–5/8   10–2/3   10–7/12–year–old boy

Word division: If end–of–line word division is used, follow the rules for English or medical word division. If the rule is not known or is unclear, refer to a standard English or medical dictionary for guidance.

Medical words are generally divided according to word parts, i.e., prefix, root, suffix. It is preferable to divide after a prefix or before a suffix rather than within the root word.

hyper–tensive   hypo–thyroidism   hyper–lipo–proteinemia
ultra–sound   radio–immuno–assay   esophago–gastro–duodenoscopy

In general, English words are divided according to pronunciation. This is the system employed by most American dictionaries.

Do not divide words of one syllable.

through   strength

Divide words between syllables.

dis–charged   tran–scrip–tion–ist   fur–ther

Do not divide words of two syllables when one of the syllables is a single vowel.

equal   amount   above

Do not divide words of five or fewer letters.

bowel   cocci   daily   into   major   prior   upper

Avoid dividing a word before a single-vowel syllable unless the vowel is the first syllable of a word root or suffix, e.g., **able** or **ible**.

thera-pist, *not* ther-apist   remark-able

When the **a** or **i** in **able** or **ible** is pronounced with the letter(s) preceding it, divide the word after the **a** or **i.**

palpa-ble   capa-ble

When the final consonant of a verb is doubled to form the past tense or the participle, the second consonant is a part of the letters following it.

admit-ting   commit-ted

A two-letter syllable may end a line, but avoid carrying a two-letter word ending to the next line.

ad-mitted   sug-gested, *not* suggest-ed

Words containing hyphens should be divided only at the existing hyphens.

well-nourished, *not* well-nour-ished

Words compounded of other words and written as one should be divided at natural breaks.

bed-time   eye-glasses   weight-bearing   eye-grounds

A word with a prefix should be divided after the prefix rather than at any other point.

ultra-sound   intra-uterine   intra-venous   intra-muscular

Most words ending in **ing** may be divided just before the **ing.**

experienc-ing

Do not divide proper names.

Presbyterian Hospital

Avoid dividing personal names. If this is not possible, break after the middle initial or between the first and last names if there is no middle initial.

John F./Kennedy Hospital   *not:* John/F. Kennedy Hospital

Do not divide abbreviations or acronyms.

wbc's   COPD   VACTERL   VATER syndrome

Do not divide numbers.

8,600   1,500,000

Transcribe a numeric value and its abbreviation or unit of measure on the same line.

51.9 kg   49 mg%

In dates, make the division between the day and the year, not between the month and the day.

March 21,/1984   November 30,/1984

Do not separate a title from a proper name.

Dr. Dirckx   John H. Dirckx, M.D.

NUMBERS

Quantities: Except as specified below, spell out single-digit numbers (one through nine). Use numerals for numbers greater than nine. In a series including numbers less than and greater than nine, use numerals for all the numbers.

52 segs, 3 bands, 28 lymphs, 11 monos

Symbols and abbreviations: Use arabic numerals with most symbols and abbreviations.

59 segs   CO2 of 42   2+
SMA-6, SMA-12, SMA-20

Units of measure: Use arabic numerals with abbreviations of units of measure. Use the numeral or write out the number if the unit of measure is written out.

5 mg, *not* five mg   8 in., *not* eight in.   12 cc, *not* twelve cc
four cubic centimeters, 4 cc, or 4 cubic centimeters   *not* four cc

Do not abbreviate a unit of measurement used with a number that has been written out.

One percent Xylocaine with epinephrine was infiltrated. *(not:* One % Xylocaine)

Four cubic centimeters . . . *(not:* Four cc . . .)

Decimals: Precede metric quantities of less than one with a zero and a decimal to avoid their being misread as whole numbers. With whole numbers, do not add a decimal or zero to avoid their being misread as larger quantities.

Premarin 0.625 mg, *not* .625 mg
0.5 mg, *not* .5 mg
8 cc, *not* 8.0 cc

NOTE: In EKG readings, the values given are in seconds and should also have a zero placed before the decimal for clarity.

EKG: Normal sinus rhythm, rate 68, PR 0.20, QRS 0.08, QT 0.42, axis +60°.

Fractions: Use fractions to express quantities of English measure which are less than one. Decimals are rarely used with English measure, unless the fractional amount is very small. Do not use fractions with metric measure.

    4 inches, 4 in.
    15 pounds, 15 lb.
    4½ inches, *not* 4.5 inches
    0.5 mg, *not* 1/2 mg
    0.018-inch stainless steel wires

In mixed fractions, use a hyphen to separate the whole number from the fraction and a slash (/) to separate the numerator from the denominator (unless the fraction may be expressed by a single key on the keyboard).

    He increased the prednisone over the last 2-1/2 weeks (*or* 2½ weeks).

Spell out common fractions. Use a hyphen with adjectival forms, no hyphen with noun forms.

    He took one-half tablet before bedtime.
    He decreased the prednisone by one half.

Percentages: Express percents with arabic numerals. Use decimals to indicate less than one; do not use fractions with percents. Use the symbol %, if available; otherwise spell out **percent.**

    0.25% *(not 1/4%)*   1.5% *(not 1-1/2%)*

Laboratory values: Use arabic numerals to express laboratory values.

    SGOT 38   creatinine of 1.6   sed rate 5

Large numbers: Express values of 10,000 and over in the traditional manner, utilizing a comma to separate thousands from hundreds, and millions from thousands. Values from 1000 to 9999 may be expressed as dictated, or in the traditional manner.

    Dictated: white count of "sixteen thousand eight hundred"
    Transcribed: white count of 16,800

    Dictated: white count "forty-eight hundred"
    Transcribed: white count 4800, or white count 4,800

    Dictated: white count "four point eight thousand"
    Transcribed: white count 4.8 thousand, or 4,800

    Dictated: CBC "eighty-nine hundred"
    Transcribed: CBC 8900, or CBC 8,900

Dictated: "four million units of penicillin"
Transcribed: 4 million units of penicillin *or* 4,000,000 units of penicillin

Specific gravity: Express specific gravity with four digits and a decimal point, with the decimal point placed between the first and second digits. This is the only correct form, even though the value may be dictated as "ten __."

Dictated: Specific gravity "ten twenty."
or: Specific gravity "one point zero two zero."
Transcribed: Specific gravity 1.020.

pH: Express **pH** by a whole number or a whole number followed by a decimal point and one or two digits.

The pH was 4.55.

Plus and minus signs: It is preferred to use numerals with the plus (+) and minus (-) signs when expressing the strength of a response or reaction. An alternative acceptable form is to repeat the plus or minus sign the appropriate number of times. However, when the plus or minus sign is repeated, the reader must count the repetitions in order to know the degree of response. Thus, numerals are preferred.

Preferred: 4+ gram-positive cocci   Acceptable: + + + + gram-positive cocci

If the phrase "plus or minus" is dictated, this may be expressed by a single key (±) **if available** or with the symbols for plus and minus separated by a slash (+ /-).

Ratios: Express ratios with arabic numerals and colons. (See section on **Colons.**)

Mycoplasma 1:2   cold agglutinins 1:4   Zolyse 1:10,000

Chemical symbols: Use arabic numerals within chemical symbols. Type the numerals on the same line as the letters, unless the keyboard provides smaller-sized numerals for use in subscripting. This facilitates reading chemical symbols because the numbers are not squeezed between two lines of single-space typing; it also eliminates the possibility of the numerals being misread as superscripts on the next line, or being missed altogether. Do not place a hyphen between the letters and numerals within a chemical symbol.

CO2   O2   FeSO4   HCO3

Express mass numbers with chemical symbols as follows; the third example requires a keyboard with smaller-sized numerals for superscripting:

I-131   or   iodine 131   or ^{131}I

Vitamins: Use arabic numerals with vitamin designations. It is preferable to type the numeral on the same line as the letter, unless the keyboard provides a smaller-sized numeral for use in subscripting. Do not place a hyphen between the letter and the numeral.

vitamin B1, vitamin B_1 vitamin B12, vitamin B_{12}

Blood pressure: Express blood pressure readings with numbers and the use of the slash. Include "mmHg" to express millimeters of mercury if dictated; it is optional otherwise.

    blood pressure 158/78   blood pressure 158/78 mmHg

Temperature readings: Express temperature readings with arabic numerals and decimal points. Add the degree sign or the word **degrees** and F or C (Fahrenheit or Celsius) if dictated; they are optional if not dictated. If the keyboard provides the degree sign (°), it is preferable to use it rather than writing out the word **degrees.**

    35.4° *or* 35.4°C *or* 35.4 degrees
    98.6° *or* 98.6°F *or* 98.6 degrees

Apgar score: Use arabic numerals to express the Apgar score of an infant. The Apgar score evaluates the infant at one and five minutes in terms of heart rate, respirations, color, muscle tone, and response to stimuli.

    Apgars were 4 and 8 at one and five minutes.

Compound nouns: Use numerals in compound nouns which include a number. Join the numeral and noun with a hyphen.

    alpha–1   profile–1   SMA-12

Drug dosage and instructions: Use numerals to express strength, volume, dosage, and directions for drugs.   Exception: The number one (1) may be written out or expressed as a numeral, unless it is followed by an abbreviated unit of measure, at which time the numeral should be used.

    8 units NPH
    20 mEq of KCl
    Lactulose 30 ml p.o. q.6h.
    E.E.S. 400 mg one q.i.d. x 5 more days
    Pen-Vee K 500 mg q.i.d. for 10 days
    Theo-Dur 200 every 8 hours or 300 every 12 hours
    Beclovent 2 puffs q.i.d.
    Valium 15 mg q.i.d. x 2 days
    Robitussin 1 tsp. q.4h.
    Hydrodiuril 50 mg daily
    Procardia 10 mg every 8 hours
    Nalfon 300 mg one q.4h. p.r.n. inflammation
    Neosporin ophthalmic solution 2 drops q.i.d. x 3 more days

When translating b.i.d., t.i.d., q.i.d., q.4h., q.6h., etc., use numerals or write out the numbers.

    b.i.d., twice a day, *or* two times a day, *or* 2 times a day
    t.i.d., three times a day, *or* 3 times a day
    q.i.d., four times a day, *or* 4 times a day
    q.4h., every four hours, *or* every 4 hours
    q.6h., every six hours, *or* every 6 hours

With eponyms: Use roman numerals to number eponymic titles.

Billroth I anastomosis, Billroth II anastomosis

With type and factor: Use roman numerals to number types and factors.

type II hyperlipoproteinemia, type IIb hyperlipoproteinemia
factor VIII (blood clotting factors)

Suture sizes: Stainless and nonstainless steel sutures are sized by the USP system. Sizes range from 11-0 (smallest) to 7 (largest). Sizes #1 through #7 are expressed as whole numbers. Sizes 0 through 0000 may be expressed by the appropriate number of zeros or in the "digit hyphen zero" format (1-0, 2-0, 3-0, and 4-0). Suture sizes 5-0 through 11-0 should use the "digit hyphen zero" format to avoid the necessity of the reader counting zeros to determine suture size.

Stainless steel suture sizes may also be sized by the Brown and Sharp (B & S) gauge. B & S sizes are expressed in whole numbers from #40 (smallest) to #20 (largest).

Cranial nerves: While roman numerals are preferred, arabic numerals may be used to number the cranial nerves.

cranial nerves II through XII (*or* II-XII)
cranial nerves 2 through 12 (*or* 2-12)

Vertebrae and intervertebral spaces: Use arabic numerals to number vertebrae and intervertebral spaces.

C7	T12	L3	S1

L5-S1
L4-5 (*or* L4-L5)

With gravida, para, ab: While arabic numerals are preferred, roman numerals may be used in expressing the obstetrical history of a patient.

gravida 3, para 2, ab 1
or:
gravida III, para II, ab I

Classes of heart disease: Use arabic numerals to classify heart disease.

functional class 2

Cardiac murmur grades: While arabic numerals are preferred, roman numerals may be used to grade cardiac murmurs.

grade 2/6 *or* grade II/VI

EKG leads: Use roman numerals for limb leads, arabic numerals for chest leads.

limb leads I through IV
chest leads V1 through V6

Cancer stages and grades: Use roman numerals for cancer stages, arabic numerals for cancer grades.

stages I through IV   grades 1 through 4

Visual acuity: Use arabic numerals to express visual acuity.

20/100   20/200

Dates: Use arabic numerals to express the day of the month and the year. Write out the name of the month; do not identify the month by a number or abbreviation. Use four digits to express the year; do not abbreviate.

March 9, 1984   9 March 1984   September 1984

not: 3/9/84   3-9-84   Mar. 9   Sept. 1984   March 9, '84   September '84

Ordinals: Spell out single-digit ordinals (first through ninth); express ordinals of greater than ninth as numerals (11th, 12th, etc.). Do not use ordinals for the day of the month if the year is given.

He was seen on the first of March and began Cytosar on the 25th.
He was seen on March 20, 1984, not March 22nd as previously stated.

Age: Ages one through nine may be written out or expressed with numerals. Use numerals with ages ten and over. Use numerals with fractions.

age 50
an 8–5/12–year–old male
a 54–year–old black female
8 years old *or* eight years old
3–year–old female *or* three–year–old female
7–1/2–year–old female, *or* 7½–year–old female

Units of time: Write out the numbers one through nine when used with units of time that are spelled out (years, months, weeks, days, hours, minutes, seconds), and use numerals for values over nine. Use numerals if an abbreviation is used for the unit of time. Use numerals if the quantity contains a mixed fraction. See previous rule for expressing ages.

five days   three minutes   48 hours
10 days   q.6h. or q. 6 h.   2-1/2 or 2½ hours
one- to two-year history   eight hours prior to discharge

Use numerals with a.m. and p.m. (AM and PM), placing a colon between the hours and the minutes. For whole hours joined with a.m. or p.m., add the colon and zeros if used in proximity with other times for which the minutes are given; otherwise they may be omitted. Use **o'clock** only with whole hours, writing out the hour or expressing it as a number. Never use **o'clock** with a.m. or p.m. Express locations utilizing time (in operative reports) as dictated. In expressing military time (the 24-hour clock), use four digits, including zeros if necessary and omitting the colon.

8:15 a.m., *not* 8:15 o'clock

four o'clock or 4 o'clock   0400 and 1830 hours

Their appointments are at 4:00 and 4:15 p.m., respectively.

The technicians drew 8 a.m. and 4 p.m. blood sugars.

Incision was made at 8:30 o'clock.

At beginning of sentence: Do not use a number at the beginning of a sentence. Instead, insert an appropriate word, e.g., "a," "an," or "the"; recast the sentence; or write out the number if its usage permits.

Dictated: 82-year-old Caucasian male was admitted.
Transcribed: This 82-year-old Caucasian male was admitted.

Dictated: 6-8 Hz waves predominated
Transcribed: Waves of 6-8 Hz predominated.

Dictated: 48 hours after admission the rash had cleared completely.
Transcribed: Forty-eight hours after admission the rash had cleared completely.
        or: The rash had cleared completely 48 hours after admission.

Dictated: 24 hours after admission the patient became clammy.
Transcribed: Twenty-four hours after admission the patient became clammy.
        or: The patient became clammy 24 hours after admission.

One percent Xylocaine with epinephrine was infiltrated.

Ties of 2–0 silk (at beginning of sentence), *not:* 2–0 silk ties

A #114 Teflon-tipped catheter, *not:* #114 Teflon-tipped catheter

Numbers together: When two numeric quantities are side by side, spell out the one more easily or appropriately expressed in words, or recast the sentence.

potassium chloride 20%, one tsp. t.i.d. in water or juice
or 20% potassium chloride, 1 tsp. t.i.d. in water or juice
two 4 x 4 cotton pledgets
Apgars were 4 and 8 at one and five minutes.

Series: Use arabic numerals to number items in a series. In series numbered vertically, follow the number with a period, capitalize the first letter of each numbered entry, and end each entry with a period to demonstrate it is complete.

ADMITTING DIAGNOSES:
1. Migraine.
2. Cervical outlet syndrome with radiculitis.
3. Chronic anxiety.

In series numbered horizontally, i.e., within a paragraph, enclose each number in parentheses.

> ADMITTING DIAGNOSES: (1) Migraine, (2) cervical outlet syndrome with radiculitis, (3) chronic anxiety.

Plurals: Form the plural of numbers by adding **s,** with no apostrophe.

> Blood sugars in the low 100s were noted.

Symbol x: In phrases such as the following, use the symbol **x** for "times," followed by a space and then the appropriate arabic numerals.

> Urine culture showed no growth x 2.

> The patient received Cerubidine 120 mg daily x 3 on the 26th, 27th, and 28th; he received Cytosar 200 mg IV over 12 hours x 14 doses beginning the 26th; and thioguanine 80 mg in the morning and 120 mg in the evening for a total dose of 200 mg a day, starting the 26th x 14 doses.

The symbol **x** may also mean "by" when used in dimensions.

> The specimen measured 2 x 1 x 4 cm.

> Two 4 x 4 cotton pledgets were used.

Number symbol (#): Use the symbol # with an arabic numeral to denote the size of an instrument or suture. The symbol # may be replaced by the abbreviation **No.,** although the symbol is preferred. If the word **number** is not dictated, the use of the symbol # or the abbreviation **No.** is optional.

> #32 chest tube
> #7-0 Prolene
> a #114 Teflon-tipped catheter

PARENTHESES

Parenthetical information: Use parentheses to provide parenthetical information; the parentheses may or may not be dictated.

> *Parentheses dictated:* Pelvic ultrasound was read as intrauterine changes consistent with pyometria. (It is difficult to believe that this diagnosis could be made on the basis of an ultrasound.)

> *Parentheses not dictated:* Further past history shows outpatient pulmonary function tests with a forced vital capacity of 2.57 liters (that is 62% of predicted), an FEV-1 of 0.98 liters.

Place a period at the end of a parenthetical entry if it is a complete sentence and it is not placed within another sentence. (See first example above.) If the parenthetical entry is within a sentence, begin it with a lowercase letter and omit closing punctuation within the parentheses, whether or not it is a complete sentence. (See second example above.) Be sure to add the closing parenthesis even if the dictator omits it.

Medications include Flexeril for fairly chronic back pain (without neurological referral). (Physician dictated the opening parenthesis but not the closing one.)

Enumeration: Parentheses may also be used to enumerate items within a paragraph. (See section on **Periods.**) When enumerating items within a paragraph, place arabic numbers in parentheses with no periods. Separate the enumerated items by commas or semicolons.

He has a long history of known diagnoses, including (1) chronic silicosis, (2) status post left thoracotomy, (3) arteriosclerotic cardiovascular disease. He was followed as an outpatient.

PERIODS

End of sentence or phrase: Use a period at the end of a declarative sentence or a complete thought.

Lung fields were clear. Cardiac exam was unremarkable.

Heart sounds normal. Lungs clear.

Enumerations: When enumerating items one under another, use a period following the numeral. Capitalize the first letter of the first word; lowercase the other words unless they are always capitalized. Use of a period at the end of each entry demonstrates that the entry is complete.

1. Upper respiratory infection.
2. Chronic obstructive pulmonary disease.

When enumerating items within a paragraph, place arabic numbers in parentheses with no periods. Separate the enumerated items by commas or semicolons.

He has a long history of known diagnoses, including (1) chronic silicosis, (2) status post left thoracotomy, (3) arteriosclerotic cardiovascular disease. He was followed as an outpatient.

Quotation marks: Place the period within quotation marks when a sentence ends with a quotation.

He says that he believes the prednisone will eventually "kill me."

Decimals: Use the period as a decimal point.

Lanoxin 0.25 mg   albumin 3.2   bilirubin 1.9   specific gravity 1.015

Chemical symbols: Never use periods with symbols for chemical elements.

K   Na   O2   CO2

Abbreviations: Do not use periods with capitalized abbreviations or acronyms.

WBC   HEENT   PAT   EKG   FANA   PERRLA   TED

The preferred style is to omit periods in lowercase abbreviations. Exception: For abbreviations used in the dosage or directions for medications, the preferred style is to use periods.

wbc   rbc

t.i.d.   q.6h.   p.o.   q.a.m.   q.i.d.   h.s.   p.r.n.

Do not use periods in abbreviations which include uppercase and lowercase letters.

aVL   aVF   mEq   IgG   HbAg   pH

Brief forms: Do not use periods with abbreviations which are brief forms of words.

exam   ab   sed rate   prep   subcu

but: in. (not *in*) for inch

Units of measure: Never use periods with abbreviations of units of measure in the metric system. Periods with abbreviations of English units of measure are preferred but optional unless the abbreviation may be misread if the period is not used.

mg   gm   cc   ng   dl   cm   mm

in. *not* in   lb. *or* lb   ft. *or* ft

Laboratory values: When multiple laboratory results are reported, separate values of related tests by commas, unrelated tests by periods.

LABORATORY EXAMINATION: Sodium 139, potassium 4.6, chloride 106, bicarb 28, BUN 15, creatinine 0.9. White count 5.9, hemoglobin 14.6, hematocrit 43.1. PT 11.3, PTT 31.4. Urinalysis: pH 6, specific gravity 1.006, negative dipstick and negative microscopic exam. Chest x-ray revealed no acute disease. EKG: Normal sinus rhythm, rate 68, PR 0.20, QRS 0.08, QT 0.42, axis +60°.

Specific gravity: Express specific gravity with four digits and a decimal point, with the decimal point placed between the first and second digits. This is the only correct form, even though the value may be dictated as "ten __."

> Dictated: Specific gravity "ten twenty."
> or: Specific gravity "one point zero two zero."
> Transcribed: Specific gravity 1.020.

pH: Express pH by a whole number or a whole number followed by a decimal point and one or two digits.

> The pH was 4.55.

Genus: Use a period following the single letter abbreviation of a genus.

> E. coli   H. influenzae

PLURALS

There are general and specialized rules for forming plurals, as well as exceptions to these rules. When uncertain, consult a medical or English dictionary for plural forms. When the dictionary does not specify a plural form, or when specialized rules do not apply, the plural is formed in the conventional manner, i.e., by adding **s** or **es** according to the first two rules below.

Most words: Add **s**.

> fluids   symptoms   tablets

Words ending in s, x, z, ch, or **sh:** Add **es**.

> reflex, reflexes   research, researches   wash, washes

Exceptions: For some words ending in **x**, change the **x** to **c** or **g** and add **es**:

> thorax, thoraces   appendix, appendices   phalanx, phalanges   meninx, meninges

Words ending in y, preceded by a consonant: Change the **y** to **i** and add **es**.

> study, studies   biopsy, biopsies   extremity, extremities

All-capital abbreviations: Add **s**. Use of the apostrophe to form plurals is acceptable but **not** preferred.

> EOMs   WBCs   PVCs   DTRs   ABGs

Single letters, symbols, lowercase abbreviations: Add **'s.**

    wbc's   rbc's   serial K's ranged from . . .   +'s

Numbers: Add **s,** no apostrophe.

    blood sugars in the low 100s

Abbreviations of units of measurement: The plural form is the same as the singular form; do **not** add apostrophe or **s.**

    4 mg   3 cc   8 g   7 lb   2 ft   6 in.

Units of measure which are spelled out: Use the plural form.

    five milligrams   nine centimeters

Brief forms: Add **s.**

eos	monos	lymphs	segs
basos	polys	blasts	bands

Eponyms, names: Add **s** or **es;** use the **es** form if the singular form ends in **s, x, z, ch, sh.** Do **not** use an apostrophe to form the plural of a name. (If forming the plural with **s** or **es** would change the pronunciation of the singular form, make no change for the plural.)

    Babinskis were negative.
    The master patient index lists hundreds of Joneses.

Medical words derived from Latin or Greek: Form plurals according to the medical dictionary. General rules follow:

Words ending in en: Change ending to **ina.**

    foramen   foramina

Words ending in a: Add **e.**

conjunctiva	conjunctivae
sclera	sclerae
sequela	sequelae
axilla	axillae

Words ending in us: Change the ending to **i.**

coccus	cocci
embolus	emboli
fundus	fundi
malleolus	malleoli
nevus	nevi

pneumococcus	pneumococci
rhonchus	rhonchi
bronchus	bronchi

Exceptions:

| bolus | boluses |
| viscus | viscera |

Words ending in on: Change the ending to **a.**

| criterion | criteria |
| ganglion | ganglia |

Words ending in is: Change the ending to **es.**

anastomosis	anastomoses
diagnosis	diagnoses
ecchymosis	ecchymoses
metastasis	metastases
naris	nares
paralysis	paralyses
pelvis	pelves
thesis	theses

Exceptions:

| arthritis | arthritides |
| epididymis | epididymides |

Words ending in um: Change the ending to **a.**

diverticulum	diverticula
serum	sera
sputum	sputa

Alternate plural forms: Words for which there is a plural Latin or Greek form as well as an English form: use the preferred form according to the dictionary, i.e., the form listed first, unless the dictating physician prefers an alternative acceptable form. When the dictionary specifies more than one plural form, the first one listed is usually the preferred form.

gases *is preferred to* gasses

Compound nouns: For compound nouns written as one word, add the appropriate ending, usually **s.**

fingerbreadths

Compound nouns written with hyphens or spaces: Add the appropriate plural ending to the word that is the essential noun.

brothers-in-law   chiefs of staff   physicians of record   attorneys at law

Compound nouns containing a possessive: Make the second word plural.

    bachelor's degrees   master's degrees   driver's licenses

Collective nouns: The term's usage determines whether the collective noun is singular or plural. A unit of measure is treated as a singular collective noun.

    A minimal amount of bleeding was present.
    A minimal amount of adhesions were present.
    A number of subjects are experiencing positive reactions.
    The number of controls was small.
    Twenty milliequivalents of KCl was given.

Genus: Use the plural form of the genus name if there is one. When there is no plural form, add the word **organisms** to show plural usage.

    Diplococcus, diplococci   Aspergillus, aspergilli
    Campylobacter organisms   Trichomonas organisms

Singular or plural: Some words may be singular or plural in usage.

    biceps   facies   series   data

    none (may mean "not one" or "not any")

Some words are always plural in usage.

    adnexa   feces   forceps   genitalia   measles   menses   scissors   tongs   tweezers

Some words are always singular in usage.

    ascites   herpes   lues

Bruit: The plural form of **bruit** is **bruits.** The final **s** is not heard in the French pronunciation, while it is in the English. The use of the word, not its pronunciation, determines whether it is singular or plural.

    There is no bruit heard.
    There are no bruits heard.

QUOTATION MARKS

Place quotation marks around a direct quotation, coined words, or quoted phrases to which the dictator wishes to draw attention.

Place the period within quotation marks when a sentence ends with a quotation.

> She had questionable "low thyroid" many years ago.
> The ileal lumen was "slitlike" at the anastomosis.
> The patient said he fears prednisone will eventually "kill me."

SEMICOLONS

Independent clauses: Connect closely related independent clauses with a semicolon if no conjunction (e.g., **and, but, for, or, nor, yet, so**) is dictated. If a connecting word such as **however, moreover, therefore, nevertheless, besides, also, then, similarly, namely, instead,** or **rather** is used to introduce the second independent clause, a semicolon rather than a comma **must** precede the connective word. Alternatively, the independent clauses may be written as separate sentences.

> He received Cerubidine 120 mg daily x 3 on the 26th, 27th, and 28th; he received Cytosar 200 mg IV over 12 hours x 14 doses beginning the 26th.
> *or*
> He received Cerubidine 120 mg daily x 3 on the 26th, 27th, and 28th. He received Cytosar 200 mg IV over 12 hours x 14 doses beginning the 26th.

> The patient had a breast operation approximately a year ago for a malignancy of the breast; however, the nodes were negative.
> *or*
> The patient had a breast operation approximately a year ago for a malignancy of the breast. However, the nodes were negative.

> The patient was seen in consultation; the consultant suggested degenerative arthritis, left knee.
> *or*
> The patient was seen in consultation. The consultant suggested degenerative arthritis, left knee.

Series: Use semicolons to separate items in a complex series or in a series in which one or more entries contain commas. Commas may be used to separate items in a simple series or in a series in which entries do not contain commas.

> The patient was discharged on the following regimen: theophylline 15 cc four times a day; Carafate 1 gm four times a day, 30 minutes after meals and one at bedtime; bethanechol 25 mg p.o. q.i.d.; and Reglan 5 mg at bedtime on a trial basis.

> Medications: Theo-Dur 300 mg p.o. b.i.d., prednisone 30 mg p.o. q.a.m., Bronkometer 2 puffs q.i.d.

> Current regimen includes Norpace 150 q.6h., Procardia 20 mg q.6h., 20% KCl 15 cc q.i.d., digoxin 0.125 mg q.a.m., nitroglycerin paste 1-1/2 inches q.6h., Surmontil 25 mg t.i.d., nitroglycerin 0.4 mg sublingual p.r.n., and Benadryl 50 mg q.5-6h. p.r.n.

SLASH MARKS (DIAGONALS, VIRGULES)

Per: Use a slash (/) to express **per** with units of measure when there is at least one specific numeric quantity and when the element immediately on each side of the slash is either a specific numeric quantity or a unit of measurement.

When the slash is used, abbreviate the units of measurement, but when **per** is written out, also write out the units of measurement. If the unit of measurement does not have an acceptable abbreviated form, use **per** instead of a slash.

    Sed rate was noted to be 52 mm/h.

    The patient's cortisol was less than 1 mcg/dl on repeat studies.

    . . . only 1 wbc/cu mm *or* 1 wbc/mm³
    or: only one white blood cell per cubic millimeter

    Pulse was increased to 120 beats per minute.

    The patient consumes approximately three bottles of wine per day.

Over: Use a slash to present values when one is dictated as "over" the other.

    blood pressure 150/80
    reflexes 2+/4+
    grade 2/6 holosystolic murmur

Fractions: Use a slash to express a fraction if a single-key fraction is not available on the keyboard. Use single-key fractions only if they are available for all the fractions in the series.

    2-1/2
    5-7/16
    21-2/3
    2½ and 2¼ *but:* 2-1/2 and 2-5/8

Ratio: Do not use a slash to express a ratio. Use a colon.

    cold agglutinins 1:4   *not:* 1/4

    Zolyse 1:10,000   *not:* 1/10,000

    Mycoplasma 1:8   *not:* 1/8

Plus or minus: Use a slash to express **or** in the phrase **plus or minus**. Alternatively, some keyboards have a single key for the symbol ±.

    +/-   ±

SPELLING

The cardinal spelling rule in medical transcription is to verify the spelling in an acceptable dictionary or other reference. **Never** accept the spelling offered by the dictator (or anyone else) unless you already know it is correct. Although the dictator's spelling of a word is not considered definitive until verified through authoritative sources, the suggested spelling is very helpful to the medical transcriptionist in finding the correct spelling and is always appreciated.

For lists of words commonly misspelled in medical transcription, see the **Appendix,** pp. 57-60.

References: Desk-size recommended English dictionaries include *Webster's Ninth New Collegiate Dictionary* and *The American Heritage Dictionary. Webster's Third New International Dictionary of the English Language* is a recommended unabridged dictionary.

Full-size recommended medical dictionaries are *Dorland's Illustrated Medical Dictionary* and *Stedman's Medical Dictionary.* Ancillary medical dictionaries include *Taber's Cyclopedic Medical Dictionary, Blakiston's Gould Medical Dictionary,* and *Encyclopedia and Dictionary of Medicine, Nursing, and Allied Health.*

Consult the **Bibliography,** pp. 61-63, for complete citations of dictionaries, word books, and other specialized references for use in medical transcription.

Alternate spellings: Some words, English and medical, have more than one acceptable spelling. In such cases, either may be used, with the selection determined either by the dictating physician, the employer or supervisor, or the medical transcriptionist. To determine the preferred spelling, consult the dictionary.The spelling which accompanies the meaning of the word is preferred. Secondary spellings are those which direct the reader to another (preferred) spelling in order to find the meaning. Example: Dorland's prefers *disk* to *disc,* and *curet* to *curette.* Webster's prefers *gray* to *grey.*

When there is a discrepancy between spellings given by the medical dictionary and the English dictionary, use the medical spelling. Example: Dorland's gives no alternate spelling for *distention;* Webster's offers *distension* or *distention.* The preferred form in medical reports, then, is *distention.*

While **disk** and **disc** may be used interchangeably (with the **disk** spelling being preferred), it is necessary to consult the dictionary to determine which spelling form serves as the root word when a suffix is attached.

    diskectomy, *not* discectomy
    discogenic, *not* diskogenic

While **curet** and **curette** are alternate spellings (with the **curet** spelling being preferred), the double-t form must be used when spelling word forms derived from the root word.

    curetting, curetted, curettage

The words **obtain** and **attain** may be used interchangeably in describing achievement of hemostasis. Transcribe as dictated.

> Hemostasis was obtained.   *or:*   Hemostasis was attained.

The noun and adjective forms of certain words are pronounced the same but spelled differently. Use the adjective form when the term describes another noun, the noun form when the word functions as a noun.

> Mucous membranes are clear.
> Clear mucus was seen in the vaginal canal.

Plural spelling: Use the general rules to form plurals unless the dictionary provides the plural form. When the dictionary provides more than one plural form, the first one listed is usually the preferred spelling. (See also the section titled **Plurals.**)   Example: Webster's prefers *gases* to *gasses*.

Word parts: Occasionally a prefix or suffix is used as an independent word.

> Abdomen: There is no **megaly.**
> **Lysis** of adhesions was carried out.

Anatomic features: It is common practice to mix the English and Latin names of anatomic parts, i.e., using English for the noun and Latin for the adjectives.   It is acceptable to transcribe these as dictated.

> latissimus dorsi muscle   palpebrales mediales arteries
> peroneus profundus nerve   temporales profundi veins

SYMBOLS

Plus and minus signs: The symbols for plus (+) and minus (–) may be used to express the rhesus factor of blood type. Alternatively, the word "positive" or "negative" may be written out.

> Rh positive *or* Rh +
> blood type O negative *or* blood type O–

The plus or minus sign may also be used to indicate a response or reaction. It is preferred to use numerals with the plus and minus signs to indicate the strength of the response or reaction; alternatively, the plus or minus sign may be repeated the appropriate number of times. Since the latter style requires that the reader count the repetitions in order to know the degree of response, the use of numerals is preferred.

> Preferred: 4+ gram-positive cocci
> Acceptable: ++++ gram-positive cocci

The phrase **plus or minus** is represented by a single-key symbol (±) on some keyboards. Alternatively, use a slash (/) to express **or** in the phrase **plus or minus** (+ /-).

Symbol x: In phrases such as the following, use the symbol **x** for "times," followed by a space and then the appropriate arabic numerals.

> Urine culture showed no growth x 2.
> The patient received Cytosar x 14 doses.

The symbol **x** may also mean "by" when used in dimensions.

> The specimen measured 2 x 1 x 4 cm.
> Two 4 x 4 cotton pledgets were used.

Number symbol (#): Use the number symbol (#) with an arabic numeral to denote the size of an instrument or suture. The symbol # may be replaced by the abbreviation **No.,** although the symbol is preferred. If the word **number** is not dictated, the use of the symbol # or the abbreviation **No.** is optional.

> #32 chest tube   #7-0 Prolene   a #114 Teflon-tipped catheter

Percent sign (%): Use the symbol (%) or spell out **percent** when a number accompanies the word. Do not space between the number and the symbol.

> 0.25%   1.5%   5%   10 percent

> The percent of patients who recover . . . (*not:* The % of patients . . .)

Greek letters: Use symbols for Greek letters if the keyboard provides them. Otherwise, write out the English translation of the letter.

> alpha   beta   delta   gamma

Ampersand (&): Avoid using the ampersand (&) except in phrases containing abbreviations separated by **and.** Do not space before or after the ampersand.

> D&C   dilatation and curettage
> T&A   tonsillectomy and adenoidectomy

UNDERLINING

In medical reports a dictator may instruct the transcriptionist to underline certain words, phrases, or sentences for emphasis. When directed to underline content, underline the content continuously including spaces and punctuation marks, except the final punctuation mark.

> She drinks probably more than the normal amount of alcohol.

APPENDIX

Spelling: Words commonly misspelled in medical transcription.

accommodation
aggravated
albumin
ambulant
aminophylline
anticoagulant
anulus
apparent
aphthous
appendiceal
ascites
assessment
asthma
asymmetrical, asymmetry
auricular
bolus
brawny
breath, breathe
bruit, bruits (plural)
cafe au lait
claudication
coccidioidomycosis
compatible
consistent
control, controlled, controlling
Coombs' test
Crohn's disease
curvilinear
decrescendo
defer, deferred
defervesce, defervescence
dependency, dependent
descensus
desiccated, desiccation
diabetes mellitus
diaphoresis
diarrhea
discogenic
Dyazide
dyspareunia
dyspnea, dyspneic
ecchymosis, ecchymoses
effusion

emittance
emphysema
en bloc
encroachment
en masse
Escherichia
exacerbation
exquisite
extraocular
extreme
facies
fatigability
felon
flu
fluctuance
fluorescence, fluorescent
funduscopic
gallop
gauge
guaiac
Haemophilus, Hemophilus
hemoptysis
Homans' test
infarct, infarction
inflamed, inflammation, inflammatory
intact
intermittent
in toto
Kerley B lines
laryngeal
liquefaction
maneuver
Morison's pouch
murmur
nicking (arteriovenous)
nitroglycerin
normocephalic (*not* normal cephalic)
occasional
occur, occurred, occurring
ophthalmic, ophthalmology
palpitation
parenchymal
paroxysmal

peau d'orange
perfusion
persistent
pharyngeal, pharynx
phlegm
plaque, plaquing
plain (film of the abdomen; *not* plane)
pneumonia
precede, preceding
predominance, predominant
primigravida
prominence, prominent
protrusion
protuberant
pruritus
psychiatry
pterygium
purulent
recumbent
recur, recurrence, recurrent, recurring

reducible
refer, reference, referral, referring
regimen (of drugs, *not* regime)
relief
rhythm
sequela, sequelae
shocky
shotty nodes
spleen
subsided
subtle
supplementation
swaged (swaged-on sutures)
symmetrical, symmetry
syncope
telangiectasis
transferred, transferring
Trendelenburg
Weber test
xanthelasma

Similar words frequently confused in medical transcription.

ab-, ad-
abduct, adduct
aberrant, afferent, efferent, inferent
abscess, aphthous
accept, except
access, assess, excess, axis
adenocyst, adenosis
advice, advise
a febrile course, afebrile course
affect, effect
affective, effective
agonist, antagonist
air, ear
allusion, elusion, illusion
an adequate, inadequate
angle, ankle
anisocoria, anisophoria
ante-, anti-
anterior, interior, inferior
anuresis, enuresis
aphagia, aphasia
apophysis, epiphysis
apposition, opposition
arrhythmia, erythema, edema
a symptomatic, asymptomatic
assess, access, excess, axis

atopic, atrophic, ectopic, atoxic
attain, obtain
a traumatic, atraumatic (injury)
Auer, hour, our
aural, oral
axis, access, assess, excess
bare, bear
beer, Bier
bloc, block
cardia, cardiac
carotene, creatine, creatinine, keratin
caudate, chordate, cordate
chondroma, condyloma, chordoma
chord, cord
choreal, chorial, corneal
chromal, clonal
cirrhosis, psoriasis
cite, site, sight
claustrum, colostrum
coarse, course
complement, compliment
complementary, complimentary
concussion, convulsion
condyloma, chondroma, chordoma
conscience, conscious
convulsion, concussion

Cooper's ligament, Poupart's ligament
cor, core, corps
cord, chord
corneal, choreal, chorial
council, counsel
course, coarse
creatine, creatinine, carotene, keratin
cystitome, cystotome
cytoblast, cytoplast
decent, descent, dissent
decision, discission
defuse, diffuse
diaphysis, diastasis, diathesis
die, dye
diffuse, defuse
dis-, dys-
discreet, discrete
dosage, doses
dye, die
dys-, dis-
dyskaryosis, dyskeratosis
dysphagia, dysphasia
ectopic, atopic, atrophic, atoxic
edema, erythema, arrhythmia
effect, affect
effective, affective
efferent, afferent, aberrant, inferent
efflux, reflux, reflex
elicit, illicit
emanate, eminent, imminent
embrocation, imbrication
eminent, imminent, emanate
enervation, innervation, denervation
ensue, ensure
enuresis, anuresis
err, error, air, heir, hair, hear, here
erythema, arrhythmia, edema
exacerbation, exasperation
except, accept
excess, access, assess
facial, fascial
facies, feces
fascial, facial
fatal, fetal
feces, facies
fetal, fatal
fissure, fistula
flail, frail
flange, phalangeal
flexor, flexure

frail, flail
fundal, fungal
furuncle, caruncle, carbuncle
gate, gait
gauge, gouge
hair, heir, air, err, error, hear, here
hour, Auer, our
hyper-, hypo-, hydro-
hypophysis, hypothesis
ileum, ilium
illicit, elicit
imbrication, embrocation
imminent, eminent, emanate
in-, en-, an-
inadequate, an adequate
induction, introduction
inertia, insertion
infarction, infraction
inferent, afferent, efferent, aberrant
inferior, interior, anterior
infra-, intra-, inter-, intro-, infero-
innervation, enervation, denervation
insertion, inertia
insight, in situ, ascites
install, instill
insufflate, insulate
integrate, integument
intralocular, intraocular
inferior, anterior, interior
introduction, induction
it's, its
keratin, carotene, creatine, creatinine
knead, need
knuckle, nuchal
lacerate, macerate, masticate, masturbate
laryngeal, pharyngeal
larynx, pharynx
lavage, gavage
lean, lien
led, lead
lichen, liken
local, lochial
loop, loupe
loose, lose
loss, lost
macerate, lacerate
macrocytosis, microcytosis
malleolus, malleus
marital, martial
masticate, masturbate

medial, mesial
melenic, melanotic
metacarpal, metatarsal
metaphysis, metastasis
miner, minor
mitigate, militate
molding, moulding
mucous, mucus
myeloma, myoma
near, Neer
need, knead
nuchal, knuckle
nucleide, nuclide
obtain, attain
opposition, apposition
oral, aural
oscheitis, osteitis
osteal, ostial
osteitis, oscheitis
ostial, osteal
our, hour, Auer
packed, pact
pair, pare, pear
palpation, palpitation, papillation
para-, peri-
parenteral, parental
pare, pair, pear
pass, passed, past
peace, piece
pear, pair, pare
pedal, petal
perfusion, profusion, protrusion
perineal, peroneal, peritoneal
perineum, peritoneum
petal, pedal
phalangeal, flange
pharyngeal, laryngeal
pharynx, larynx
phlegm, phlegmon
piece, peace
plain, plane (plain film of abdomen)
plaque, plague
pleural, plural
Poupart's ligament, Cooper's ligament
pray, prey
precede, proceed
prey, pray
principal, principle
proceed, precede

procession, progression
profusion, perfusion, protrusion
prostate, prostrate
psoriasis, cirrhosis
pump, sump
pylorus, pyosis
pyogenic, pyrogenic
pyosis, pylorus
pyrogenic, pyogenic
raise, raze, rays
rail, rale
rate, wait, weight
recession, resection
reflex, reflux, efflux
regimen, regime, regiment
residence, residents, resonance
resolution, revolution
reticulum, retinaculum
revolution, resolution
root, route
sac, sack
scatoma, scotoma
scent, sent, cent
sight, site, cite
sprain, strain
stationary, stationery
sump, pump
talipes, telepathy
telepathy, talipes
their, there, they're
through, thorough, threw
tic, tick
track, tract, tracked, trachea
trichinosis, trichocyst, trichosis
uncal, uncle, ungual
ureter, urethra
ureteral, urethral
valgus, varus
Verres, Voorhees
vertex, vortex
vesical, vesicle
viscous, viscus
Voorhees, Verres
vulva, uvula, uvea
waist, waste
wait, weight, rate
waive, wave
weight, wait, rate
your, you're, yore

BIBLIOGRAPHY

Accreditation Manual for Hospitals. Chicago: Joint Commission on Accreditation of Hospitals, 1984.

The American Heritage Dictionary. 2nd college ed. Boston: Houghton Mifflin Co., 1982.

Barr, Janice K. "Editing Practices—An Overview," in *Journal of the American Association for Medical Transcription* 2, no. 3 (Fall 1983):12-13.

Baumann, Joyce. "The Many Faces of Editing in Medical Transcription," in *Journal of the American Association for Medical Transcription* 2, no. 3 (Fall 1983):14.

Bates, Barbara. *A Guide to Physical Examination.* 3rd ed. Philadelphia: J. B. Lippincott Co., 1983.

Bennett, Kathy. "An Introduction to Editing," in *Journal of the American Association for Medical Transcription* 1, no. 1 (Summer 1982):38-39.

Bennington, James L. *Saunders Dictionary & Encyclopedia of Laboratory Medicine and Technology.* Philadelphia: W. B. Saunders Co., 1984.

Berris, Kyle. "Pharmaceutically Speaking," in *Journal of the American Association for Medical Transcription* 3, no. 1 (Spring/Summer 1984):32-34.

Billups, Norman F., and Shirley M. Billups. *American Drug Index.* 26th ed. Philadelphia: J. B. Lippincott Co., 1984.

Birk, Newman P., and Genevieve B. Birk. *A Handbook of Grammar, Rhetoric, Mechanics, and Usage.* Indianapolis: The Bobbs-Merrill Co., 1972.

Blackburn, Janice. "The Editing Department," in *Journal of the American Association for Medical Transcription* 1, no. 1 (Summer 1982):39-40.

Blakiston's Gould Medical Dictionary. 4th ed. Novato, Calif.: McGraw-Hill Book Co., 1979.

Blauvelt, Carolyn Taliaferro, and Fred R. T. Nelson. *A Manual of Orthopaedic Terminology. St. Louis:* The C. V. Mosby Co., 1981.

Brown, Lin. "Editing in a Teaching Hospital," *in Journal of the American Association for Medical Transcription* 1, no. 1 (Summer 1982):41.

Buchanan, Robert E., and Norman E. Gibbons. *Bergey's Manual of Determinative Bacteriology,* 8th ed. Baltimore: The Williams & Wilkins Co., 1974.

Cassin, Barbara, and Sheila Solomon. *Dictionary of Eye Terminology.* Edited by Melvin L. Rubin. Gainesville, Fla.: Triad Publishing Co., 1984.

Chabner, Davi-Ellen. *The Language of Medicine.* 2nd ed. Philadelphia: W. B. Saunders Co., 1981.

The Charles Press Handbook of Current Medical Abbreviations. 2nd ed. Philadelphia: The Charles Press Publishers, Inc., 1984.

The Chicago Manual of Style. 13th ed. Chicago: The University of Chicago Press, 1982.

Coleman, Frances. *Guide to Surgical Terminology.* 3rd ed. Oradell, N.J.: Medical Economics Co., 1978.

Covel, Sue. "Balancing Quality with Quantity," in *The Best of AAMT,* 1982, American Association for Medical Transcription, p. 20..

Covel, Sue. "President's Message—Uniform Standards: Are They Necessary for Medical Transcription?" in *Journal of the American Association for Medical Transcription* 2, no. 2 (Summer 1983):3.

Current Medical Information & Terminology. 5th ed. Chicago: American Medical Association, 1981.

Current Procedural Terminology. 4th ed. Chicago: American Medical Association, 1983.

Diehl, Marcy Otis, and Marilyn Takahashi Fordney. *Medical Typing and Transcribing: Techniques and Procedures.* 2nd ed. Philadelphia: W. B. Saunders Co., 1984.

D'Onofrio, Mary Ann. "Transcribing for the ESL Physician," *Journal of the American Association for Medical Transcription* 1, no. 1 (Summer 1982):36-37.

Dirckx, John H. *The Language of Medicine: Its Evolution, Structure, and Dynamics.* 2nd ed. New York: Praeger Publishers, 1983.

Dorland's Illustrated Medical Dictionary. 26th ed. Philadelphia: W. B. Saunders Co., 1981.

Dunmore, Charles W., and Rita M. Fleischer. *Medical Terminology: Exercises in Etymology.* Philadelphia: F. A. Davis Co., 1977.

"Editing Practices in Medical Transcription," edited by Sally C. Pitman, in *Journal of the American Association for Medical Transcription* 1, no. 1 (Summer 1982):38-46.

Ellis, Barbra. "The Medical Report—A Shared Responsibility," in *Journal of the American Association for Medical Transcription* 2, no. 3 (Fall 1983):6-7.

Equipment/Instrument Reference List. Seattle: Transcription Services, University of Washington Hospital, 1983.

Facts and Comparisons. St. Louis: J. B. Lippincott Co., 1984.

Fischbach, Frances. *A Manual of Laboratory Diagnostic Tests.* 2nd ed. Philadelphia: J. B. Lippincott, 1984.

Follett, Wilson. *Modern American Usage: A Guide.* New York: Hill and Wang, 1966.

Fowler, H. W. *A Dictionary of Modern English Usage.* 2nd ed. revised by Sir Ernest Gowers. Oxford: Oxford University Press, 1965.

French, Ruth M. *Guide to Diagnostic Procedures.* 4th ed. Novato, Calif.: McGraw-Hill Book Co., 1975.

Fuller, Joanna Ruth. *Surgical Technology: Principles and Practice.* Philadelphia: W. B. Saunders Co., 1981.

Gray, Henry. *Anatomy of the Human Body.* 29th ed. Edited by Charles Mayo Goss. Philadelphia: Lea & Febiger, 1984.

Guerrero, Arlean. "Abbreviations: A High-priced Convenience," in *The Best of AAMT,* 1982, American Association for Medical Transcription, p. 21.

Guerrero, Arlean. "Quality Vs. Quantity," in *The Best of AAMT,* 1982, American Association for Medical Transcription, pp. 16-17.

Harrell, Jean. "Communication Through a Medical Document," in *Journal of the American Association for Medical Transcription* 2, no. 3 (Fall 1983):18.

Horn, Patricia. "Editing Physician Dictation," in *Journal of the American Association for Medical Transcription* 2, vol. 3 (Fall 1983):5.

Horn, Patricia. "Practicing Editing Skills," in *Journal of the American Association for Medical Transcription* 1, no. 1 (Summer 1982):44.

Horn, Patricia. "Punctuation: The Vital Link," *Journal of the American Association for Medical Transcription* 1, no. 1 (Summer 1982):34-35.

Huffman, Edna K. *Medical Record Management.* 7th ed. Berwyn, Ill.: Physicians' Record Co., 1981.

The International Classification of Diseases. 2nd ed., Clinical Modification. Washington, D.C.: U.S. Department of Health and Human Services, 1980.

Jetchick, Gayle. "A Survey of Editing Practices," in *Journal of the American Association for Medical Transcription* 1, no. 1 (Summer 1982):45.

King, Lester S. *Why Not Say It Clearly: A Guide to Scientific Writing.* Boston: Little, Brown & Co., 1978.

Lorenzini, Jean A. *Medical Phrase Index.* Oradell, N.J.: Medical Economics Co., 1978.

Magalini, Sergio, and Euclid Scrascia. *Dictionary of Medical Syndromes.* Philadelphia: J. B. Lippincott, 1981.

Manning, Ruth. "A Novice Looks at Editing," in *Journal of the American Association for Medical Transcription* 2, no. 3 (Fall 1983):10-11.

Manual for Authors & Editors: Editorial Style & Manuscript Preparation. 7th ed. Compiled for American Medical Association by William R. Barclay, M. Therese Southgate, and Robert W. Mayo. Los Altos, Calif.: Lange Medical Publications, 1981.

Marshall, Judith. "Birds of a Feather," in *Journal of the American Association for Medical Transcription* 1, no. 2 (Winter 1982-83):48; "Card Sharks," *JAAMT* 2, no. 1 (Spring 1983):48.

Marshall, Judith. "Tape Dancing," p. 15, and "What Is a Medical Transcriptionist?", p. 14, in *The Best of AAMT,* 1982, American Association for Medical Transcription.

Medical Abbreviations Handbook. 2nd ed. Oradell, N.J.: Medical Economics Books, 1983.

The Merck Manual. 14th ed. Rahway, N.J.: Merck Sharp & Dohme Research Laboratories, 1982.

Michaels, Davida., ed. *Diagnostic Procedures: The Patient and the Health Care Team.* New York: John Wiley & Sons, 1983.

Miller, Benjamin F., and Claire Brackman Keane. *Encyclopedia and Dictionary of Medicine, Nursing, and Allied Health.* 3rd ed. Philadelphia: W. B. Saunders Co., 1983.

Mosby's Medical Speller. St. Louis: The C. V. Mosby Co., 1983.

Nomenclature and Criteria for Diagnosis of Diseases of the Heart and Great Vessels. 8th ed. Boston: Little, Brown & Co., 1979.

Physicians' Desk Reference. 38th ed. Oradell, N.J.: Medical Economics Co., 1984.

Pitman, Sally C. "Editor's Message [on Editing Practices]," in *Journal of the American Association for Medical Transcription* 2, no. 3 (Fall 1983):4.

Pitman, Sally C. (ed.). *The eMpTy Laugh Book.* Modesto, Calif.: American Association for Medical Transcription, 1981.

Pitman, Sally C. (ed.). *Journal of the American Association for Medical Transcription,* seven issues, Summer 1982-Spring/Summer 1984.

Pyle, Vera. *The AAMT Notebook.* 2nd ed. Modesto, Calif.: American Association for Medical Transcription, 1982.

Pyle, Vera. *Current Medical Terminology.* Modesto, Calif.: Prima Vera Publications, 1985.

Pyle, Vera. "A Medical Transcriptionist's Fantasy," in *Journal of the American Association for Medical Transcription* 2, no. 4 (Winter 1983-84):3.

Pyle, Vera. "A Question of Style," in *Journal of the American Association for Medical Transcription* 1, no. 2 (Winter 1982-83):11; 2, no. 2 (Summer 1983):26; 2, no. 3 (Fall 1983):38-39; 2, no. 4 (Winter 1983-84):23; 3, no. 1 (Spring/Summer 1984):10.

Ramirez, Elizabeth M. "Editing the Medical Report," in *Journal of the American Association for Medical Transcription* 2, no. 3 (Fall 1983):20-22.

Regimbal, Carole. "Problem: Quality Control in Medical Transcription. Solution: 'Consultant of the Week' Program," in *The Best of AAMT,* 1982, American Association for Medical Transcription, pp. 18-19.

Rimer, Evelyn H. *Harbeck's Glossary of Medical Terms.* Menlo Park, Calif.: Pacific Coast Publishers, 1967. (out of print)

Roe-Hafer, Ann. *The Medical & Health Sciences Word Book.* Boston: Houghton Mifflin Co., 1982.

Sabin, William A. *The Gregg Reference Manual.* 5th ed. New York: McGraw-Hill Book Co., 1977.

Shaw, Harry. *Writing and Rewriting.* 5th ed. New York: Harper & Row, Publishers, Inc., 1973.

Shortridge, Anne O. "President's Message—The Quest for Excellence: Go for the Gold!" in *Journal of the American Association for Medical Transcription* 3, no. 1 (Spring/Summer 1984):4-5.

Sloane, Sheila B. *The Medical Word Book.* 2nd ed. Philadelphia: W. B. Saunders Co., 1982.

Sloane, Sheila B., and John L. Dussau. *A Word Book in Pathology and Laboratory Medicine.* Philadelphia: W. B. Saunders Co., 1984.

Smith, Margaret. "Editing Dictation by Word Processor," in *Journal of the American Association for Medical Transcription* 2, no. 3 (Fall 1983):16.

Stedman's Medical Dictionary. 24th ed. Baltimore: The Williams & Wilkins Co., 1982.

Steen, Edwin B. *Bailliere's Abbreviations in Medicine.* 5th ed. London: Bailliere Tindall, 1984.

Stein, Harold A., Bernard J. Slatt, and Penny Cook. *Manual of Ophthalmic Terminology.* St. Louis: The C. V. Mosby Co., 1982.

Strunk, William, Jr., and E. B. White. *The Elements of Style.* 2nd ed. New York: The Macmillan Co., 1972.

Szulec, Jeannette A., and Z. Szulec. *A Syllabus for the Surgeon's Secretary.* 3rd ed. Detroit: Medical Arts Publishing Co., 1980.

Taber's Cyclopedic Medical Dictionary. 14th ed. Edited by Clayton L. Thomas. Philadelphia: F. A. Davis Co., 1981.

Tessier, Claudia. "Guidelines and Ground Rules," in *Journal of the American Association for Medical Transcription* 2, no. 3 (Fall 1983):40-41; 2, no. 4 (Winter 1983-84):29; 3, no. 1 (Spring/Summer 1984):43.

Tessier, Claudia. "Results of the 1982 Certification Examination," in *Journal of the American Association for Medical Transcription* 2, no. 1 (Spring 1983):9-14; "Results of the 1983 Certification Examination," in *JAAMT* 2, no. 2 (Summer 1983):12-18.

Tessier, Claudia. *The Surgical Word Book.* Philadelphia: W. B. Saunders Co., 1981.

Tietz, Norbert W. *Clinical Guide to Laboratory Tests.* Philadelphia: W. B. Saunders Co., 1983.

Tilkian, Sarko M., Mary Boudreau Conover, and Ara G. Tilkian. *Clinical Implications of Laboratory Tests.* St. Louis: The C. V. Mosby Co., 1983.

Voogd, Trudy. "Ghost Editing in Medical Transcription," in *Journal of the American Association for Medical Transcription* 2, no. 3 (Fall 1983):8-9.

Wallach, Jacques B. *Interpretation of Diagnostic Tests.* 3rd ed. Boston: Little, Brown & Co., 1978.

Webster's Ninth New Collegiate Dictionary. Springfield, Mass.: Merriam-Webster, Inc., 1983.

Webster's Third New International Dictionary of the English Language, Unabridged. Springfield, Mass.: Merriam-Webster, Inc., 1981.

Widmann, Frances K. *Clinical Interpretation of Laboratory Tests.* 9th ed. Philadelphia: F. A. Davis Co., 1983.

Words into Type. Based on studies by Marjorie E. Skillin, Robert M. Gay, and other authorities. 3rd ed. Englewood Cliffs, N.J.: Prentice-Hall, Inc., 1974.

INDEX

ABOUT THE AUTHORS

Claudia Tessier has been director of education of the American Association for Medical Transcription since January 1983. She has six years' experience in medical transcription, including three years with a national transcription service. Tessier has taught medical terminology and transcription in community college and adult education settings and has taught medical record administration at the University of Illinois in Chicago and the University of Wisconsin in Milwaukee. She has 12 years' administrative experience in health care and education settings and holds a master's degree in allied health education, a bachelor's degree in health education, and an associate degree in medical secretarial science. Tessier is a certified medical transcriptionist and a registered records administrator. She is also author of *The Surgical Word Book,* published by W. B. Saunders in 1981. She serves as assistant editor of the *Journal of the American Association for Medical Transcription* and contributes articles frequently, including the column, "Guidelines and Ground Rules." She has led numerous AAMT workshops on transcription practices and teaching medical transcription and has developed the AAMT medical transcription training module in general medicine to be released early in 1985.

Sally C. Pitman, as director of publications, has produced numerous educational publications for the American Association for Medical Transcription since 1979. A member of the AAMT Board of Directors for six years, she has served as chair of the AAMT certification examination committee since 1982 and has led several AAMT workshops on transcription practices and writing for publication. She has been editor of the quarterly *Journal of the American Association for Medical Transcription* since Summer 1982, editor of the bimonthly *AAMT Newsletter* since March 1979, editor of the compilation, *The Best of AAMT* (1982), and compiler/editor of *The eMpTy Laugh Book,* published by AAMT in 1981. Before she entered the medical transcription field, she worked on publications for three university presses, earned B.S. and M.A. degrees in English, completed two years of postgraduate work, and taught college English for five years. In the past ten years as a medical transcriptionist and owner/manager of a medical transcription service, she has trained many medical transcriptionists on the job. Currently she is owner of Prima Vera Publications which specializes in medical and educational publications.